Iron Chic: Adventures of an NPC body builder.

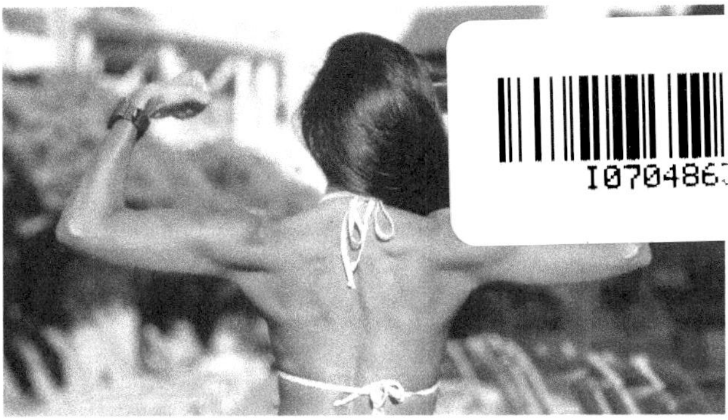

By Chaitra KR

Dedication

This book is dedicated to my incredible family, with an extra dose of enthusiasm reserved for my rock-solid husband. Your unwavering support and boundless encouragement have been the driving force behind every lift, every stride, and every milestone reached. Your belief in me has been my guiding light, propelling me forward on this exhilarating journey.

To coaches Kelly and Danny, you have turned the gym into a playground of excitement and inspiration. Your infectious energy and innovative approach made every workout a thrilling adventure. Thank you for helping me break into the world of lifting weights and for making fitness not just a routine, but a passion.

A special shout-out to Bony, my eternal source of inspiration and unwavering support. You took my aspirations and cranked them up a notch, showing me the true path to bodybuilding excellence. Through every trial and triumph, you stood tall like an oak tree, offering guidance and strength when I needed it most.

And to Coach Ty and Jo, your exceptional coaching, steadfast support, and unwavering love have been the driving force behind my NPC journey. Your dedication to teaching me the discipline required for muscle building and the importance of nutrition in bodybuilding has been invaluable. Thank you for instilling in me the knowledge and determination to pursue my dreams with passion and purpose.

With boundless gratitude and love,

Chaitra KR

Contents

Chapter 1: The Epiphany

In those nebulous days of origin, the world remained oblivious to the quiet genesis of an impending catastrophe. It unfolded clandestinely, escalating exponentially until it had ensnared our precious orb within its firm grasp – a somber symphony of suffering, disease, and death. The scourge we now confront bears the name Corona Virus, or more formally, COVID-19. Whispers in the wind suggest that its genesis was traced to the heart of China, where an unwitting protagonist unwittingly partook of a deceased bat, unknowingly infected with an insidious ailment. In the throes of their unfortunate demise, they unwittingly ushered forth a legacy destined for global proliferation. This viral entity possesses a cruelly elegant mechanism of transmission, borne upon the very breath of humanity. Its contagion is unyielding, manifesting in myriad forms, from the insidious theft of smell and taste to the affliction of one's vitality, culminating in a most dire fate - the inexorable grasp of death.

To counter this rampant contagion, we have been relegated to the confines of our own abodes. Our world, the one we once knew, has been overtaken by a pervasive pandemic. The Homo sapiens, known as humans in the common parlance, find themselves conscripted into an unwitting but vital role in the preservation of our imperiled planet - to hunker down within the sanctuary of their homes, a last bastion of safety against the unexpected march of this viral specter.

From local media, social networks, and daily news, we are continually inundated with information about the effects of the pandemic and the virus's symptoms. This repetition persists until those very symptoms manifest vicariously, like a lunatic on the loose, imploding into our minds with immense mental stress. If the Corona Virus spares your physical existence, it unquestionably ensures that you endure a daily mental ordeal within the confines of your home.

"Isolation," "Social Distancing," "Face Masks save lives," "Epidemic to Pandemic," and numerous other once-foreign concepts have now seamlessly woven themselves into our everyday discourse, carrying newfound gravity among us. As days have dwindled away in this dystopian lockdown, isolating us from the world, we have grown increasingly reliant on our digital existence for human interaction.

We are now connected with each other from our homes. Working from home privileges, along with social media platforms such as Zoom and Webex-based meetings, and yes, telephone calls, continue to dominate in this ever-changing, technologically advanced yet challenging world. Ironically, the term "new normal" swiftly found its place in the year 2020's dictionary, amidst its rapid updates. The planet, as we know it, must now grapple with the aftermath of the pandemic.

But the question that looms large is whether it will heal.

What force can take this merciless beast that exponentially ravages lives with each passing day?

By God's grace, for those of us who can endure despite the virus's far-reaching effects by staying home and working remotely, our challenges primarily consist of isolation and, at times, boredom, when considered within the broader context of the events that unfolded in the tumultuous year of 2020.

The lockdown bestowed upon us an invaluable gift – time for introspection into the lives we lead. It was, in its own way, a divine message, urging us to slow down and savor the essence of life. As paradoxical as it may seem, while the pandemic ruthlessly claimed lives, it also served as a blessing in disguise during our moments of confinement. It served as a stark reminder for us to focus on aspects we had previously neglected: the blessings and the intrinsic value of life itself.

Three months have elapsed within the confines of our homes, and it was time to redirect our focus toward these very blessings, while also affording the world beyond a chance to embark on its healing journey. At the commencement of the state lockdown, there was a palpable sense of chaos as we scrambled to stock our homes with essentials, including dry pantry goods, replenishing the fridge, securing toilet paper, and obtaining hand sanitizer. These measures were taken to ensure that we had everything necessary at our disposal, reducing the need to venture outside whenever possible.

Once our homes were adequately equipped, the subsequent step involved an extensive spring cleaning of our living spaces. With all of us restricted to our homes, the daily surplus of energy demanded an outlet, and the surplus of time provided an opportunity for productive use. This period became characterized by cleaning, organizing, streamlining, and a meticulous exploration of our dwelling. It was surprising to realize just how much we tend to accumulate within our homes, spanning from trivial miscellaneous items to absolute necessities. Yet, despite this accumulation, our desires remain insatiable, and we persist in accumulating materialistic artifacts that momentarily gratify us, entertain us, and, eventually, falsely define our sense of pride and ownership.

Once the home had been tailored to meet certain personal expectations, goals, and functionality, the focus shifted entirely to the family. The inhabitants of the household, including pets, children, spouses, aunts, uncles, grandparents, and even the chirping bird in the corner, received dedicated attention. The gift of time suddenly became available, allowing for the strengthening of relationships that had often taken a backseat due to the demands of work, careers, and the pursuit of financial success. It did not matter whether one was rich or poor, young, or old, a celebrity or a commoner, single or married; across the world, we all found ourselves adhering to a quarantined lifestyle to preserve life itself. Together, we formed an army to combat a common foe, working toward a singular goal – to conquer an invisible arch-nemesis, a virulent creature of lethal intent, whose sole purpose was to inflict harm, sow chaos through a ruthless chain reaction of infections, and, to extinguish life.

Initially, family time felt akin to being on vacation - a vacation where the rush to begin each day with mundane activities, obligations, and personal growth was replaced by the simple joys of relaxation, sleeping in, focusing on the family, engaging in shared activities, and deepening intimate bonds. The lockdown transformed our lives into a staycation, gifting us with time that was crucial in our collective effort to safeguard the world. Interactions with other individuals were rendered perilous, for anyone could unknowingly carry the deadly invisible virus that lurked in the streets.

We had an abundance of time to spend with our household members, which was profoundly fulfilling, until a yearning for a new, personally designed personal space began to emerge. Alongside this desire for expanded personal boundaries came a growing sense of confinement within the four walls of our homes.

As time passed and personal boundaries took shape, this sense of confinement evolved into a feeling of desolation, leading to a kind of internalization that drained our energies. We found ourselves, in a peculiar twist of fate, akin to animals confined within the cages of a zoo, yearning for freedom and wide-open spaces beyond our domestic confines.

Do we tread down the treacherous path of self-destruction, disrupting the delicate equilibrium of the human mind and body?

Can we harness the time that has been thrust upon us so reluctantly, seizing it as an opportunity to unearth our true callings?

As humble inhabitants of this virus-ridden planet, we may not be destined for grandiose aspirations like those luminaries who have left an indelible mark on the annals of history. Most of us are, indeed, ordinary folk, grappling with life's unpredictable twists and turns, striving to endure each passing day with as much grace as we can muster.

But let us begin this introspection with the person who gazes back at us from the mirror's reflection.

What does that individual harbor within their heart, a dream or aspiration that has been obscured by the sands of time?

Could it be that this personal goal was inadvertently consigned to oblivion, relegated to the shadows as other, more immediate concerns took precedence?

Why not seize this opportunity to rekindle those personal aspirations, to breathe new life into the dreams that may have long lain dormant?

Consider these thoughts...

I was fortunate that in the initial stages of the virus spread, I had already planned to commit to a personal goal. This goal was not only geared towards promoting my well-being but also offered the satisfaction of checking off one of the many items on my to-do list, which I had longed to accomplish before my time on this Earth concluded.

What did I choose?

Something I never thought I would dream of doing: Preparing for an NPC bodybuilding bikini competition at the State level.

Why did I consider this goal?

You may ask, or even if you do not ask, or do not care—well, the simple fact that you are reading my book obliges me to share my tale in my Iron Chic: Adventures of an NPC body builder. It is often in life's insignificant and humble pursuits that the deepest personal interests are discovered. The clock must tick, the web must weave, and thus, here is my fitness journey, replete with its challenges, in the year 2020.

My hope is that by conveying my dramatic story in the isolation of 2020, I can inspire others and highlight a goal achieved against all odds. I consider myself a physically active and restless individual. Please do not misunderstand me; I am not referring to any illness. Instead, I take pride in embodying the refined and delicate meaning of the proverb: "Movement is life."

I am, if you will, an endorphin junkie—an addict to the emotions I yearn to experience repeatedly. I can never get enough of the exhilarating rush that floods in when my opioid receptors are activated, ushering in a euphoric sense of well-being through the healthy pursuit of intentional movement, commonly known as exercise. The intrinsic factors fueling my addiction stem from the profound connection between mind and muscle.

It is in those moments when the mind harmonizes with the body, and both move in a synchrony that transcends ordinary rhythms. The mind transforms into an agent of change, propelled by the artistry of movement.

I was blessed—or some would say cursed—with a predisposition for grace and an insatiable restlessness that required movement for my very sustenance. Recognizing this unique disposition, my dear mother, bless her heart, enrolled me in a reputable classical dance school. Her intention was to channel my love for movement into a disciplined and structured art form known as Bharatanatyam, a time-honored tradition.

It is believed that Lord Shiva, the destroyer of all evil, was the creator and torchbearer of Bharatanatyam. The cosmos bore witness to his powerful dance, a gift bestowed upon humanity. The form and technique of Lord Shiva's dance were meticulously codified in a sacred text known as the Natya Shastra. This profound knowledge was then passed down to those who carried the "burden" of the necessity for movement. Humbly, I was among those fortunate souls to receive this divine treatment, a journey that commenced at the tender age of eight. Dance paved the way for a lifelong pursuit of fitness that matured with time.

Movement with grace and intention became an integral part of my identity. It often feels as though I have danced more than walked steps than I have taken while growing up. Regardless of the demands that life imposed – education, career, marriage, and motherhood – I always found time to move.

Movement coursed through my veins, serving as my sanctuary of hope and a wellspring of strength. In addition to my formal training in Indian classical dance, I consistently sought opportunities for movement throughout life—a burst of endorphins, the joyful exertion of my body, to bring balance to my mind and body amidst the routines of daily life.

I love working out for no specific reason; I simply relish the sensations that accompany it. Any form of movement induces a rush of blood to all the body's organs, liberates the muscles, and imparts a sense of mental freedom that translates into strength and control. Activating my metabolism has been the driving force behind my daily exercise routine. I have been exceptionally fortunate to have been inspired by numerous individuals I have met, connected with, and forged bonds with. I hold a deep and genuine admiration for the human body's capacity to move and flourish, offering limitless possibilities and boundless experiences through physical activity.

Eons ago, armed with only two suitcases filled with my belongings, I left my homeland, India, bidding farewell to my family and roots, and embarked on a journey across the seven seas with my knight in shining armor, my husband, to the land of the brave and the free: the United States of America.

I settled in this foreign land with the aspiration of making it my home and building a future here. Starting anew in a foreign world, every immigrant encounters the challenges of establishing their identity and security in an unfamiliar place, and it is far from an effortless endeavor.

My husband and I resided in a small apartment, leading a simple life that we made cozy, creating a home away from home. Due to limited financial resources, we embarked on our marital journey, with my husband working while I assumed the role of a homemaker. I raised my two incredible boys, instilling them with Indian values alongside American culture. Throughout the demanding and engaging years, I never lost sight of my commitment to fitness and movement.

Even on those occasions when I did lose sight of my personal pursuits due to the demands of my roles as a wife, homemaker, or a mother, my body would gently remind me of the need for movement. My nerves would twitch, offering a gentle reprimand that movement was overdue, among other aspects that required my utmost attention. If I failed to heed this internal call, I would find myself dreaming and envisioning running outdoors, feeling the wind in my hair, savoring the cool morning breeze, and basking in the rejuvenating sunrays—the ultimate source of energy.

With pent-up energy and a backlog of self-care, I felt a growing need to expend this internal reservoir; otherwise, I would feel consumed by it. Consequently, I seized any opportunity for physical activity that did not require monetary expenditure.

I utilized the gym in our apartment complex or embarked on long walks with my babies securely nestled in their baby seats, snugly positioned within a stroller that was always stocked with a diaper bag, ready for use during our extended walks.

During those precious moments when my boys were peacefully asleep, I would engage in silent practice sessions for my dance routines. These moments offered a sublime balance, a respite from the burdens of life, as my body moved to the rhythm of the music. The connection between my mind and body, liberating my muscles through movement, became an addiction that only deepened with age. As my babies grew into toddlers, I found myself constantly on the move, tending to their needs while my husband worked long hours. Movement remained an integral part of my life, even though finding time for formal exercise was challenging. I kept the inner fire burning, a flickering flame within me, serving as a constant reminder to move and experience the freedom that might one day reveal my true calling.

I fondly recall the cherished memories I created with my babies, moments of playing music in the family room, cooking in the kitchen, and even dancing with my little ones in tow. I managed to infuse movement into the midst of my family's demands and responsibilities.

After earning my bachelor's degree from an accredited state university, I embarked on my career journey. As the years rolled on and my babies continued to grow, there was never a dull moment in my life, yet I still found time for dancing whenever I could. Balancing my responsibilities and my passion for fitness took on new dimensions. Whether it was shuttling my kids to soccer practice, cross-country meets, or swim lessons, I always managed to carve out time for movement. It was during my son's YMCA swim lessons that I discovered an opportunity to attend Zumba classes, which were held simultaneously in the group fitness room.

Participating in Zumba was an incredible experience, as it allowed me to be part of a vibrant group, immersed in the collective energy that arose from the fusion of trendy music and bold movements in perfect harmony. As a classical dancer, I held a deep appreciation for all forms of art. Zumba provided a wonderful outlet that not only satisfied my desire to stay fit but also fulfilled my craving for movement.

I eagerly anticipated my son's weekly swim lessons, as they provided me with the chance to dance when he was busy. I held immense admiration for the instructor who taught the dance classes and came to realize that there was so much more to explore, learn, and adapt when it came to movement. I felt truly blessed to possess the gift and the curse of limbs that could move to the rhythm of music.

As fate would have it, the cycle of life dictates that all things, whether good or bad, eventually end. This held especially true for the stage of life I found myself in—a young mother with children, juggling various responsibilities to make ends meet for my growing family. My fitness activities were confined to brief bursts of activity, interspersed with prolonged periods of waiting, my inner fire yearning for movement. After my son's swim lessons concluded, I could no longer attend the Zumba classes, a fact that did not bother me in the least. My days were consumed by my roles as a wife, a mother, and my pursuit of a career, and I found myself once again juggling multiple responsibilities. During this whirlwind, I continued to long for the joy of dancing.

It was during this time that my son expressed a desire for the latest gaming device, the Wii, for his entertainment. Little did I know that the Wii would not only serve as a digital nanny for the kids but also fulfill my own dancing needs. I was able to purchase Zumba discs for the Wii, providing me with a similar experience in the comfort of my own home. While it could not replicate the energy and expertise of a live class with an expert instructor and fellow dancers, it sufficed to quell the constant reprimands from my body, craving movement.

Of course, practicing at home came with its own set of challenges, including my little boys running around with their toys while I attempted to dance. Many a time, our paths would collide, resulting in minor injuries for all involved. I adapted, as all human beings do. I turned it into a game for my children. I explained to them that there was an invisible circle around me, and they could not come inside it, but they were free to move around it while I practiced. The result was fantastic; injuries became less frequent, and we all had a wonderful time. As my boys grew up, there was less need for nurturing in that regard. It is fascinating to observe the natural laws that govern our existence, especially in the context of my fitness passion. Dance and movement were integral aspects of how I channeled my internal nervous energy, providing the equilibrium I sought within myself. It was not until later that I truly grasped the importance of healthy eating. I had yet another opportunity to learn something new that would alter the course of my actions. Despite considering myself active and healthy, I had never paid proper attention to my diet. I tended to skip meals and sometimes go about my day without eating. Such unhealthy eating habits, when prolonged, can have serious repercussions as one ages. With age came increasing levels of tiredness and fatigue. It is neither a myth nor magic that the energies and desires you project into the world can have a boomerang effect, with invisible forces returning those energies to you. I had believed that age and the limitations of my limbs would eventually slow me down in terms of my movement needs. Just as I was beginning to accept these biological constraints, another opportunity for change presented itself—a chance to alter the trajectory of my actions.

This opportunity arose at my workplace, which had an in-house gym. The catalyst for change was an announcement I happened upon one day. My friend and colleague Donna stated that the gym was open to all employees of the company with a free pass valid for one month. While I knew I did not have the time or the financial resources to invest in a gym membership, the allure of a free pass was undeniable. In September 2017,

I decided to join the gym to take advantage of this one-month complimentary pass.

Upon entering the gym, I was immediately overwhelmed by the array of machines, each appearing imposing and intimidating. It was a bustling lunch hour, and the gym was filled with all sorts of fitness enthusiasts. There were muscular individuals lifting dumbbells, and I could not help but wonder why they were called "dumbbells." Other highly fit individuals were diligently working their limbs using various machines. The gym members were engaged in peculiar, repetitive movements that coincided with the rhythmic "cling and clang" of weights attached to an intricate pulley system, moving up and down to an unfamiliar beat. While I was well-acquainted with the movements of my own body and limbs, this was my first glimpse of the human body in motion, manipulating external objects for strength.

There were other gym members, primarily women, clad in neon leggings or shorts paired with matching tank tops and matching headbands to keep the enormous mane in control or a high raise ponytail that bounced to an unknown rhythmic beat along with colorful athletic shoes, eagerly making their way toward a group room with a clear sense of purpose. The gym's surround sound system blasted energetic tunes, while mounted televisions displayed news or fitness-related channels. The wide windows allowed ample natural light to flood the gym area. Surrounded by people of varying backgrounds, all striving for gains or working toward goals I knew nothing about, I felt like an outsider without a clear purpose. In my newfound environment, I swiftly climbed onto the nearest treadmill.

Upon examining the treadmill's digital control panel, I was uncertain about which buttons to press to initiate its operation. I pressed a few buttons randomly, and eventually, the treadmill's conveyor belt began to move.

"Oh good, now I can walk for a while and blend in," I thought to myself.

The pace on the treadmill initially felt incredibly slow, so I decided to experiment by pressing a few more buttons. To my surprise, I discovered that I could adjust the pace, incline, intervals, and various other settings. Realizing that I needed to get comfortable with the treadmill before potentially making a spectacle of myself, I focused on adjusting the pace. I settled for a 3.0 speed, and it felt quite nice; my legs warmed up, and I was comfortable. Once I had established my rhythm on the treadmill, I casually observed the bustling gym around me. My gaze shifted to the overhead television, and I mindlessly watched the news as time passed. After twenty minutes, the treadmill had recorded a mile of walking, and I felt a sense of accomplishment for making productive use of my office break. Feeling rejuvenated, I returned to my desk and continued working for the remainder of the day.

For the next week, I stuck to the same routine. I did not feel comfortable branching out; I was shy and hesitant. I did not want to risk stumbling or making mistakes and feeling embarrassed in front of the determined individuals who frequented the gym. However, after a week had passed, my curiosity about the formidable machines in the main area of the gym got the best of me. I summoned the courage to approach Kara, the gym instructor.

She was clad in black knee-length leggings paired with a dry-fit shirt that had "coach" written on the back. Her appearance exuded fitness and strength, and she greeted me with a cheerful attitude and a warm smile. As our conversation unfolded, I found myself asking surprisingly irrelevant questions.

"Hi, I just joined the gym during this free month," I began.

"Welcome," she replied.

"Can you wear shorts in the gym?" I inquired.

"Yeah, of course!" she responded.

"Cool, I would like to work on my stomach area," I blurted out, instantly regretting my words. I had been cautious not to make a fool of myself during my time at the gym, but now I was asking the coach silly questions. In response, she kindly explained, "Workouts are structured in a way that we can't solely focus on one specific part of the body. While we do have ab workouts, it's important to think of the gym experience as a total body workout."

I tried to absorb what she had said, but my internal embarrassment made it difficult to fully grasp her explanation. The concept of a "total body experience" left me puzzled and inquisitive. What exactly did it entail? "Why can't I work on my abs? Is there no hope for me to get fit in the abdominal area after two pregnancies?" I wondered aloud. Realizing that I needed to approach my questions more cautiously, I continued, "Okay, can you help me understand how to use these machines?" My hope was that we would eventually discuss ab workouts.

"Of course," she replied, "you can schedule one-on-one sessions with either Dave or me. We can assist you with using the machines and designing workouts tailored to your needs."

"Okay, that sounds good," I responded.

We walked over to her glass-enclosed desk, where she sat down and began flipping through a large file. She carefully scanned the time slots and then proceeded to sign me up for personal training. As I left work that day, I felt enthusiastic about the prospect of personal training and a desire to learn. In the subsequent weeks, a transformation began in my fitness lifestyle with my formal introduction to the gym. Personal training marked the beginning of a new chapter in my fitness journey, one that involved utilizing various machines and iron equipment.

During my personal training sessions with the gym coaches, I maintained an elevated level of focus. I absorbed valuable insights into the significance of proper form and technique while working on different muscle groups using machines, equipment, and dumbbell weights. Lifting weights was an entirely different form of repetitive movement to which I was unaccustomed, and I found myself intrigued to learn and adapt. It was not long before I started attending more scheduled personal training sessions to become familiar with weightlifting techniques. During these sessions, I quickly realized how weak my arms and legs were when attempting to lift even the smallest weights. The coaches advised me to focus on form and technique, assuring me that lifting heavier weights would come with time as my body-built endurance and muscle.

The only association I had with muscle building was Mr. Olympia and Arnold Schwarzenegger. In my childhood years, I had seen Arnie's pictures in magazines and was fascinated by his Greek god-like physique. I had always associated muscles with men, and it never occurred to me that it could be something for women. Furthermore, I knew my free pass would expire in a month, so I did not worry too much about my initial weakness in weight training.

I concluded that women might appear too masculine if they lifted weights, a belief that was reinforced by the fact that I mostly saw men using the machines, while women dominated the group fitness rooms. With this consensus in mind, I shifted my attention to group sessions, which were primarily attended by women, with a few men. I felt more comfortable being among my peers.

The group sessions were much more enjoyable and aligned with the movement style of fitness I was accustomed to through dancing. These sessions were like a gold mine, catering to everyone's needs. There were group sessions ranging from one hour to as short as fifteen minutes. Since I was new to the gym and had limited time, I initially attended the shorter breakout sessions before and after office hours. I relished the experience of working out, bonding with fellow office workers, and networking in these sessions.

The outcomes of each session, whether they lasted an hour or just ten minutes, began to work wonders on my body, enhancing my strength and boosting my confidence. My days began with enthusiasm, as I sprang out of bed with energy, and they ended with restful sleep. The gym sessions and the variety of movements offered a refreshing change from my usual dance routines with the Wii. As a result, my body started to undergo transformation, even though my eating habits remained unchanged.

I no longer felt fatigued when climbing stairs; in fact, I had the energy to tackle them two steps at a time. Throughout the day, I felt consistently energized to move around at work, allowing me to focus on completing my tasks and deliverables in a timely manner.

My attitude and confidence improved significantly at work. I used to be seen as a quiet individual who blended into the office decor, often keeping my head down, deeply engrossed in my work, and labeled as an introvert. However, I noticed a change in myself as I started becoming friendlier and more approachable to my colleagues. My confidence was growing in ways I had never imagined. On the home front, just when I had thought my age was taking a toll on my energy levels, I suddenly became incredibly active. I embraced family life with renewed vigor, and a general sense of well-being prevailed.

I began to venture beyond my comfort zone, which had primarily been the treadmill. The gym was no longer an intimidating place; it had transformed into a space I eagerly wanted to be a part of. I felt that I had achieved a more positive and fulfilling life with the introduction of the gym. As the expiration date of my free month-long membership approached, I made the decision to become a paid member of the gym at my office. While I still did not have an abundance of time for self-care due to my work demands, the gym's programs catered to my needs.

With my newfound commitment to fitness and the positive changes I was experiencing, I decided to take it more seriously. I printed out the group session schedules and posted them on my desk's whiteboard. This allowed me to plan my gym sessions effectively, coordinating them with the demands of my workweek. I decided to give the pre-lunch twenty-minute workout a try. As I entered the group exercise room, I followed the coaches' instructions, stumbling through the routines, occasionally getting confused with right and left directions, and adjusting my pants and tee-shirt along the way. Despite the initial challenges, I managed to complete the 20-minute workout. Over the weekend, I made the decision to invest in some quality workout clothes, just like the confident women I had observed in the gym. I also purchased a good pair of workout shoes.

Having been an Indian Classical Dancer for most of my life, I had always trained to dance barefoot and never owned proper athletic attire or shoes. With a gym bag containing my new shoes stored under my desk at work, I was prepared to make fitness a regular part of my routine. I began incorporating the 20-minute workouts into my daily schedule, and I felt rejuvenated, sharp, and highly alert when I returned to my desk to continue working for the rest of the day.

As days passed, I started to opt out of my occasional outdoor walks with friends outside the office building. I eagerly looked forward to the 20-minute workouts every day. I had become so comfortable with this new fitness regimen that I loved what it was doing for my overall well-being. I wanted to share my progress and enthusiasm with others around me, so I began asking my coworkers if they were members of the gym. If they were, I would enthusiastically rave about the benefits of the 20-minute workouts and try to encourage them to try it.

On the home front, my older son was excelling in cross country at his high school. My husband, inspired by the positive effects of running, started running alongside my son to support him and prepare him for state-level cross country championships. As a dedicated father, he conducted online research to discover how to help our son increase his pace, understand the necessary dietary requirements, and appreciate the importance of rest. Running quickly became the central topic of conversation in our household. Our discussions revolved around terms like mileage, VO2 max, pace, interval training, and the superiority of running over other forms of cardio. Unfortunately, in my men's eyes, dancing held little importance, and they considered my group sessions, which focused on cardio with minimal use of weights, as less significant.

To participate in these conversations, I would share details about my gym experience and my dance practice at home, emphasizing the importance of fitness. While my men did listen to me, I always had the impression that they did not regard dancing as a legitimate sport for fitness. Moreover, I had not achieved any significant milestones in their eyes. While they were running miles, getting fit, and growing stronger with a competitive goal, I was busy cooking in the kitchen, attending to the needs of my younger child at home, and participating in the twenty-minute workout sessions at work.

During these conversations, I attempted to be more descriptive by explaining exercises like "This" and "and then this" to them. However, I often received looks as if to say, "Okay, let's get back to talking about athletics."

On weekends, my husband and my son would engage in arm wrestling matches to demonstrate their strength and discuss it. I wanted to join in too, but every time I did, I failed miserably. I realized how weak my arm strength was. Despite having excellent cardiovascular strength from years of dancing and movement, I had nothing to show in terms of physical strength.

My younger son expressed interest in participating in these friendly arm-wrestling matches, so I thought I would try wrestling with him instead. To my utter astonishment, I failed at arm wrestling my ten-year-old boy. Adding insult to injury in a house full of men, I began to struggle with tasks like taking out the trash from the kitchen to the garage, and it was even more challenging to lift it into the trash bin. I had to rely on my men to handle this task for me, and I felt like I was losing their respect or was I losing respect for myself and my capabilities?

In a desperate attempt to regain their respect and to prove to myself that I am strong, I decided to join them in running over the weekends. However, my knees began to hurt so badly that I could not even walk afterward. I was left wondering why I was losing my physical strength.

The twenty-minute sessions were not enough, or perhaps I was getting older, or it could be that my diet was not right. I was not sure why I was experiencing this sudden relapse, especially considering that I did not have extra time due to my family duties.

What should I do?

I felt grateful when an opportunity presented itself once more, and my prayers were answered. My older son's cross-country training required early morning practices on Fridays. This meant I had to drop him off at the dark hour of 5:30 am and then head to work. Fortunately, I could attend the one-hour morning classes at my office gym! Even better, Fridays were dedicated to ab workouts, which gave me a chance to see if there was any hope of shedding the family-pack of abdominal muscles I had developed over the years. Achieving a six-pack had become a dream after becoming a mother and carrying around the stretch marks and wrinkled skin from delivering two boys into this world, which I proudly accepted but often kept hidden under loose clothing. This opportunity initially only existed on Fridays, but it soon started sporadically appearing on other workdays when I had to drop my son off at his school for practice, giving me more chances to attend longer gym sessions in addition to the midday twenty-minute workouts that I never missed.

Most of the morning classes revolved around strength and resistance training, which meant lifting weights like dumbbells. I was apprehensive about lifting weights and did not want to become overly muscular, but I was eager to gain some strength, as age was starting to weaken me. I had goals in mind – I wanted to achieve milestones like my men, earn respect, and even beat my younger son in arm wrestling. With those goals in mind, without thinking much about weight training, I began attending all the morning sessions.

The routine was going well, but the more I trained, the more fatigued I felt. I started to relapse, and it seemed like I was even weaker than before I started regular gym sessions.

What am I doing wrong again?

Yet another opportunity arose to address this setback. The coaches informed me that they would be conducting sessions on nutrition and the importance of protein in the diet.

Maybe focusing on my diet will help!

The webinars on the importance of nutrition conducted by the coaches were eye-openers and came at just the right time for my fitness journey to continue. It felt like the universe was working in my favor, signaling that my fitness journey would persist. I gleaned many valuable insights on the significance of nutrition, portion sizes, and cultivating a healthy relationship with food. I decided to incorporate these lessons into my daily routine to see if they would work for me.

Primarily, to thrive and excel in strength training, I needed to increase my protein intake in my daily diet. Being a vegetarian all my life, my protein sources included eggs (which I did not particularly like), nuts, dairy, Greek yogurt, tofu, almond and peanut butter, and chickpeas. Additionally, there were protein supplements available in the form of plant protein powder, whey protein powder, and protein bars. The new rule was that every meal had to contain some form of protein, accompanied by a generous serving of colorful vegetables. The variety in colors ensured a diverse intake of nutrients to fuel the body. Carbohydrates were essential for energy, so every meal needed to include a substantial amount of carbohydrates.

I must admit, I had never paid so much attention to food until now. Previously, food had merely been a means to sustain me throughout the day, and my food choices were often influenced by my husband's preferences. Whatever he wanted, I would cook and eat, regardless of whether I liked it or not. I began to introduce one egg a day, increased my vegetable, dairy, and nut intake in every meal, irrespective of portion sizes. These changes in my meals had some impact on the energy and strength I was lacking for my resistance training. Consistency and portion control were the keys that I had failed to recognize in this new endeavor, and eventually, the demands and responsibilities of juggling my career and family life would pull me down repeatedly.

However, my desire to elevate my fitness to the next level was unwavering despite my busy schedule. The burning desire persisted, reminding me that somehow, somewhere, things would work out. I knew deep down that I had a problem with my diet. Many years of bad eating habits, including skipping meals, were something I struggled with repeatedly, even though I had attempted to discipline my eating habits on numerous occasions.

I became leaner and leaner to the extent that the doctor recommended not losing more weight. I was putting in a lot of effort to eat right and never lose sight of my training regimen, which included weights, cardio, dance, and whatever I set my mind to. I attended every single morning class, whether it was with Kara or Dave's sessions. I drew inspiration from their strength and showed them what I could do. Witnessing my progress, they began to challenge me more, and a robust symbiotic relationship developed. Days and months passed by, and I grew stronger. Not only could I beat my 10-year-old in arm wrestling, but I could do much more. My attitude toward life underwent a transformation, and my wardrobe shifted from dainty summer outfits to jeans and sneakers so I could quickly go from my desk to the gym for a workout.

The addiction to movement only intensified with age, despite not strictly following a diet and having an ab area that still resembled a family pack rather than a six-pack. I began to put on weight in the right places and lose it in the wrong places. I felt invincible and proud. I was addicted to the gym to the point that even on my days off, I would drive all the way to attend the morning class before starting my day. There were times I visited the gym at least three times a day to work out. I craved increasingly; it was like a healthy addiction, a great new drug.

I developed newfound respect for the coaches, who provided inspiring and challenging workouts that transformed me inside and out for the better. I was a completely different person, and I took immense pride in that. The entire gym experience had become a total body experience, and at last, I understood the concept of the "total body experience."

I even achieved a major milestone I had been working toward by attending numerous classes and displaying dedication at the gym. I was recognized as the Health and Wellness Fitness Ambassador for the year 2018. My poster, featuring my favorite fitness quote, adorned the hallways of my workplace near the entrance to the gym. This was my most significant accomplishment, and I was grateful for the skilled guidance of my coaches.

On the home front, my husband began investing his precious time in fitness. After transitioning from running, he shifted his focus to weight training by becoming a member of the neighborhood gym. He started lifting weights, undergoing a transformation, and fostering a positive perspective on the love for movement. The feelings and aftereffects of working out are so contagious that they make you want to keep experiencing increasingly of that sensation. These positive feelings do not stop there. Once you begin to reap the mental and physical benefits, the impact is immeasurable. Health improves, and your mental state of mind takes a positive turn.

The conversations at home revolved around fitness, and now I was able to contribute with my valuable feedback as well. My family respected my milestone, and I had my stance once more. I soon began to arm wrestling with my younger one repeatedly until he started to wail that he wanted to win. The mother in me would relent.

The more fitness talk we had, the more interesting and competitive it got with my husband and me. He invested in a year-long personal training program with a coach at his gym and began spending more time and energy at the gym than at home. As usual, all the work at home required my attention. I was used to it; that is the Indian cultural aspect that we have adapted from our parents back in India. I was a living epitome of living in a household where the man works to bring home the bread and the woman also works to bring home the bread and cook and clean it up after dinner.

I had transformed and maintained my fitness through diet and exercise, and I continued to do so without any other specific goals or intentions. Meanwhile, my husband began to transform as well and improved his diet to the extent that he gained a lot of muscle and started looking very buff and strong.

With strength comes confidence, and with confidence comes self-care and affirmation. The topic of our discussions at the dinner table and other times focused on fitness, weight training, different muscle groups and protein intake, and soon we began to have heated discussions about whose diet and workout regime was superior. Physically, his transformation was more evident than mine, so he always had an upper hand in our discussions. Diet was my weakness and time was not in my favor when I had to juggle work, kids, and home, and since I was a vegetarian, my choices of protein were limited compared to my husband's diet, which included meat, which was the problem? My husband and I became even more competitive, arguing that his workouts were better than mine, hence the difference in our transformations.

I was not offended by my husband's perspective. I knew I had diet issues, but I also knew that I had tried everything possible with fitness and believed I was better than him in that regard. When his transformation, clean eating, and healthy diet resulted in the emergence of his six-pack abdominal muscles, I became very jealous. I thought it was unfair that he did not have to go through pregnancies to have damaged-looking abdominal muscles like I did. This led to discussions about me using pregnancy as an excuse and the belief that I could show six-pack abdominal muscles if I pushed harder with my fitness regime.

Curiosity played a significant role in these discussions, more than emotional turbulence, so I decided to join my husband's gym to see what all the fuss was about. I was stumped when I entered the gym in my neighborhood. The number of machines and equipment was overwhelming, and my thirst for fitness grew even more. Meeting my husband at the gym three times a week became a romantic date and quality time for us. We supported each other through the weight training experience. We also talked, laughed, discussed our boys, and connected with each other during the one hour that we spent at the gym. Our relationship strengthened, and a year passed by.

It was time for my older son to move out to attend college. As devastating as it was to learn to live with the growing void of my son, whom I thought would stay with me after eighteen years of living together as a family, I was wrong. Nothing felt good anymore; I missed him terribly, felt lost, insecure, and destroyed. However, my younger son reminded me that he needed to eat and that my role as a mother was not yet done.

I focused on my younger boy's development, his needs, and his wishes. Slowly, the void became something I could live with and bear. I looked forward to my college son's weekend visits, which helped me see him, nurture him with loads of cooking and affection, and send him off on Sunday evenings with an icebox filled with home-cooked meals. Days and months passed, and I realized that I still had a good chunk of time on my hands now that my boys were grown up. I invested my time in more self-development through movement. This felt weird because, while raising a family, I had forgotten all about myself, my needs, my aspirations, my goals, and dreams. I was blessed to be a member of two gyms, one at work and another near my home. I was active every day, lifting weights, running, kickboxing, and soon I started attending group sessions in the neighborhood gym.

The Universe has a way of playing with needs and desires, and I am thankful for the events that followed. One of the classes I attended in my neighborhood gym was called Strong Nation, a form of workout introduced by the Zumba home office. Strong Nation was a contemporary form of HIIT (High-Intensity Interval Training), a workout where every move had a beat, and every beat had a move. The custom-created music was powerful, and so was the technique of the strong moves.

All the moves incorporated kickboxing and martial arts techniques, and with the music effects, I felt like a Ninja. I was so attracted to this form of workout that I became a licensed and certified Strong Nation instructor. Through Strong Nation, I expanded my circle of friends and found a new horizon. I connected with everyone who shared the same passion as I did. I was amazed by some of the very seasoned instructors I met and the limits they could push themselves to in terms of their cardiovascular health. I felt like I had just scratched the surface in my fitness journey. There is so much to do when you have the desire and drive to excel in everything you undertake, especially when you have the gift of time.

I continued with weight training in both gyms and a whole lot of cardio training, but my abdominal muscles still did not show. I was on the verge of accepting the harsh reality that I might never achieve my goal of visible abdominal muscles when an opportunity presented itself again, and of course, I grabbed it. I did not think much about setting goals until I met a friend at work who played a pivotal role in my fitness journey, pushing me to take the next step. Her name is Bony, and she is a sweet, quiet person who had migrated from Venezuela. I knew her as an acquaintance, a friend of a friend whom I would simply acknowledge in the hallways or the breakroom at work.

One day, I happened to be browsing for new friends on Facebook and came across Bony's profile picture. I clicked on the picture and was taken to her profile, where I saw her proudly posing with a totally fit, bronzed body in a bikini on stage and she had six pack abdominal muscles! I was taken aback and could not reconcile the picture with the person I had known in real life. Bony was an introvert, incredibly quiet and soft-spoken. In fact, I realized I had never really heard her speak. I looked at more of her album pictures and was fascinated by her stage photos. I was intrigued and decided that I would have a chat with her.

The next day, I looked for her, and at the first opportunity I had, I approached her.

"Hi, bony," I said.

"Hi," she responded with a feeble voice.

"Hey, I wanted to ask you something. I happened to come across your profile on Facebook, I guess due to a mutual friend of mine. You are a bodybuilder?"

She responded, "Yes," and she smiled, and her face lit up. That was the beginning of a beautiful, empowering friendship. We got to talking after the brief conversation, and it is so intriguing when two people find a topic of mutual interest or something they are passionate about that the friendship just clicks!

The months flew by as I talked to Bony about her fitness journey, her diet, and her experiences. I was absorbed in learning from her with every fiber of my being. She explained to me that bodybuilding was a sport, a whole other industry with an extremely strict and regimented diet and exercise program. Through our conversations, texts, and instant messaging, our friendship was blossoming. I learned so many aspects from her, starting from what macro meals (measured combination of carbohydrates, fats and protein) were and what they do for successful weightlifting and muscle building.

I was exposed to an extraordinarily rich human story and the success of her fitness journey. The more she told me, the more I wanted to know, and the more I wanted to try it out. At that point, I had tried everything from cardio and weightlifting to group classes, and I had excelled in learning to be a good instructor with Strong Nation HIIT workouts. I thought I had transformed into a healthy middle-aged woman, and I was proud of my milestones, even though I had never seen my abdominal muscles, and I thought I never would. Then Bony told me she had a six-year-old daughter.

I was astounded. How was this possible? She had gone through pregnancy like I did, but in her stage pictures, she was showing her six-pack abdominal muscles.

What I thought I knew about fitness was about taking a whole new level with my new friend. I directly asked her, "Is it possible for me to get abs like you?"

She replied, "Yes, with bodybuilding prep."

I asked, "What do you do in a body building prep?"

"Oh, it's a carefully regimented heavy-duty training of cardio, weightlifting, and eating a well-planned diet."

"And you get a six-pack?"

"Yeah." She said.

There was still hope on the horizon to see my abdominal muscles and to win in the unknown and not formally discussed competition with my husband. I began explaining all that I had achieved and done so far with my fitness.

"I want to do this prep," I declared.

Bony asked, "Do you lift weights?"

"I'm a beginner. I do lift weights, but not so much."

"Then I suggest you lift weights regularly for at least a year before committing to bodybuilding prep," Bony advised.

I replied, "Well, I do lift weights at both gyms, but I don't want to look manly with muscles."

She chuckled and reassured me, "Ha-ha, you will not look manly at all. Besides, it takes years to develop muscles. Do not worry about that; just keep lifting.". Her mantra of "Keep Lifting" stayed playing in my head from that day onwards.

I was curious that this lady was talking about a different concept of fitness of which I was not aware. Curiosity got the better of me, and I wanted to shadow her and learn about her training methods. That weekend, I printed a free pass for the gym she was a member of and shadowed her. We worked on isolation machines for legs, and we got to talk and connect through it all. We took pictures and then hung out for lunch afterward. I was enthralled by her; she was a single woman and kept herself together so well. I wanted to be like her: bold and beautiful.

However, I was not sure if I was ready to commit myself to bodybuilding prep of diet and exercises, given everything going on in my world and my family. Moreover, it was culturally wrong for an Indian woman to flaunt her physical body in a two-piece bikini, let alone on a stage in front of the world in a competition. I did not think I was ready for it, but I was glad to shadow her and learn from her. I was slowly shedding my inhibitions about lifting more in my workout regimes, even though from time to time, I wondered if I would become like those women with huge muscles. The media had ingrained that image in me with its passive aggressiveness. I wanted to avoid transforming into one, which was a significant factor in not eating or venturing into weightlifting extremes. I realized how delusional my thought process was.

Around the same time, my gym sessions with my husband took a whole new level. He had completed a year-long personal training program with a certified coach, and now it was time to be introduced to the bar, aka the barbell, and everything turned upside down. All my beliefs and notions about being fit, looking lean, and staying feminine went out the window.

Barbell workouts were a whole different ball game indeed. There were push, pull, and leg workouts scheduled on different days, along with minimal steady-state cardio. The reasoning behind such a stark demarcation of muscle groups was to isolate them and work with barbells and machines to tear those tiny muscle fibers at the gym. These muscles would later recover and regrow, producing more muscle with the right amount of protein intake outside the gym. I began to learn that a minimum of twenty-four to forty-eight hours was required for the recovery of the muscle groups worked before working them again.

With sets of a certain number of reps, these muscles in the body tend to break down, recover, and grow stronger. It was now a science with weightlifting that I began to follow along with my husband's routine. My diet and metabolism went all topsy-turvy, and I started eating a lot because I was burning a lot of calories. My delusion that weightlifting makes women huge faded into the horizon. I still remember the first month I worked out over the weekend with my husband at the squat rack; we went to Chipotle and stuffed ourselves with food. Later, I slept like a corpse for five hours in the afternoon to recover. My metabolism was alive, and I had begun to rev up from within. I started to feel stronger, more powerful, and more resilient with my body and recovery. I found myself skipping two steps and sprinting up the stairs, and I could even run outdoors with my son and my husband without experiencing knee pain. What is more exciting is that my body began to curve tiny baby biceps and triceps began to form, my shoulder cups looked like curvy cups and most of all my quads and hamstrings began to develop at a snail pace.

I could easily take out the trash with one hand now. I was strong with the introduction of the bar, and despite being inconsistent with my macros, I was still not very consistent with food intake and began eating whatever I found around me. Transformation took on a whole new level. I began filling out, looking rounder and curvier, although my abdominal muscles were still the same, a family pack. The barbell truly raised the bar for me and opened a world of possibilities. I continued my regimen at the office gym and the local gym, and soon, I started to see my body transform. I was bulking up with muscle, and it looked good on me. I was changing mentally once more. I had shape, size, curvature, and most importantly, strength within, making me capable of handling anything the world had to offer. Instead of looking like a manly female, I started to look like a healthy, fit female.

My appetite increased. Protein bars, protein powder, eggs, and healthy foods like salad, nuts, edamame, and a slew of other nutrient-rich foods became my friends. Not just for me, but even for my family; we all started eating well, eating healthily, and looking more fit, fuller, and stronger. The energy was contagious, not just at the gym; it flowed into my workplace and at these times were when I managed to accomplish to learn new technologies, obtain various management certifications that helped my job and added skills to my resume and most importantly I was not afraid to take on new tasks and responsibilities and excel in everything I put my hands on. From being an introverted caterpillar, I burst from my cocoon and flew like a beautiful curvy butterfly to new horizons. This was also the time when I reached the pinnacle of my career in terms of responsibilities, growth, and personal reviews. My attitude, my fortitude, my gait, and my personality cranked up a few notches. I was always the working mother, scrambling from morning to night, but now I was still a working mother, able to do it all from morning to night. There was no sign of relapse like I had experienced in the past. Talk about perspective! From being underweight, I put on twenty-five pounds in a span of twelve months. I was able to do all sorts of acrobatics. Nothing hurt; in fact, I had bursts of constructive collaboration, and I felt as if I was an embodiment of self-possession and solidity. I was a supermom with a cape, juggling work, home, kids, and their activities, and still having a smile at the end of the day. The age of 40s was rocking! Life was perfect.

But then human nature is such that you tend to look for challenges, a drive, and inspiration to keep going. I was not able to commit to anything apart from what was already going on in my life. My boys were grown up, and there was no one-on-one nurturing needed. It was the time during the 2020 summer holidays, and my family and I were planning to go to India for vacation. We were excited to see our respective family and friends. My husband and I were looking for flights, available dates, and working on getting approval from the office for time off. We had not seen our respective extended families for three years, and it is always good to go back home to them on vacation.

It was early February when we started to shop for deals on airfares. This was when we first began to observe the news about the Coronavirus that erupted in China and was slowly spreading to major parts of Europe. China and Italy were hit hard with the contagious virus. At first, we did not pay much attention, but soon we came to the realization that all the flights from America to India had at least one layover in Europe, and currently, European flights were being reduced or canceled due to the virus.

Nevertheless, we kept waiting and shopping, and the news media started exploding with reports about the virus, how many infections had occurred, and how fast it was spreading from China to other countries. The turn of events surely got our attention, although at that point, America was on the other side of the world, and we felt safe, or at least that was what we thought. After much deliberation, my husband and I decided to call off the India trip due to the epidemic in those countries. At that point in time, I had an epiphany to compete in a bodybuilding competition since we were not traveling. Considering that time was a gift and in lieu of travel cancellations, I took the opportunity to pursue my goals.

I decided, and that very decision carved the experiences in my fitness journey, goals, and achievements. I took a day off from work and visited Bony's bodybuilding coach at Total Fitness Gym. I walked in with uncertainty of what I would encounter. There were a lot of people in the gym working out. They all looked muscular, resilient, and tattooed. A much muscular lady with extremely broad shoulders was nearest to the door through which I entered. I reflected that I had come a long way in my fitness journey. From being completely, a gym outcast to now lifting weights without any inhibitions, I felt ready to compete.

"Hi, I have an appointment with Jo today," I said.

She pointed me to the kitchen where I had to sit. I waited and waited, and I could hear laughter, grunts of people lifting weights, and muffled conversations trickling from the gym room that was adjacent to the kitchen. A beautiful tall woman with rippling muscles came to greet me. She was dressed in gym leggings and a tank top. Her long dark hair was tied high into a ponytail. Through her sleeveless tank top, her muscles and curves on the arms were very predominant and pumped. Her long lustrous dark hair was touching her extraordinary slim waist. Her upper body was jacked, and her exposed ab area showed me the abdominal muscles that I have been in pursuit of for years now; really, she had a lot of muscle, unlike anything I had seen in my other two gyms.

"Hi, I am Jo," she said, and soon another even more magnificent male came in to shake my hand. "Hi, I am Ty," he said. I shook hands, suddenly feeling smaller and more intimidated in the presence of this powerful duo who would be my coaches for the months to come.

The coaches were happy to know that I was recommended by Bony.

"Bony is my inspiration, and I wanted to be like her, so I would like to compete in a bodybuilding competition," I said.

The consultation was based on my commitment: a clean macro-based diet that consisted of carbs, fat and protein which must be measured and followed strictly. Biweekly physical check-ins where my weight and body fat percentage would be recorded and monitored with the aid of calipers at the studio to ensure that I am on track with my diet and workouts to increase muscle mass and decrease body fat percentage. A promise and a commitment of doing cardio three times a week and weightlifting four times a week and taking a day off for rest. Another silly but a sure promise to commit to sending pictures of meals to the coaches before every meal to get the coaches approval and blessing for five weeks so that they know that I am not cheating on the meals and I am adhering to the strict discipline of eating every three hours in a day for the next twenty-five weeks, as I was a first-time bodybuilder. An hour had passed so quickly that I did not realize it at all. I walked out of Total Fitness with a whole new perspective on fitness goals. Yes, I committed to bodybuilding and preparing for competition. I had my measurements taken, my body composition analyzed, and a custom meal plan that I needed to follow for the next six months was to be given by the end of the day. I had a purpose, a calling...

My workout regime consisted of fasted cardio of running in the mornings.

Weightlifting included a clear-cut dedicated days for various muscle groups that I had to focus on with the intention of sculpting the parts of the body to build it...thus body building.

Monday - Legs (leg extension, dumbbell squats, lunges, seated, step up on bench)

Tuesday - OFF

Wednesday - Shoulders (shoulder press, dumbbell side laterals, front raises)

Back (one arm dumbbell rows, low row pulley, wide grip pulls downs)

Thursday – OFF

Friday - Legs (lying leg curls, reverse lunges, sumo squats, adductor, deadlifts)

Saturday - Chest (incline press, incline dumbbell flies. pushups,)

Arms (barbell curls, hammer curls, tri push down, dips)

Sunday – OFF.

I had to set alerts to have BCAAs pre and post workouts and a whole load of over-the-counter supplements like Omega 3, flaxseed oil, multivitamins and so on.

What changed was the meal plan that I had to follow strictly for at least six months or until my coach felt I was ready to compete! The journey was just the beginning. I took the printout of my meal plan to make a grocery list. I had never paid much attention to what I ate. I was trying to eat clean and healthy foods, which comprised eating one egg a day, making the plate rich in all colors, eating yogurt, protein powder, and indulging in sweet treats every so often. Not to mention, I had days where I did not eat much at all and simply starved because I was not hungry.

I thought that I had tried it all and found a comfortable diet that I could sustain. I felt proud that I had it all under control. I was in for a massive surprise when I created my grocery list. I had to eat much more food, specific food, and with much more specific discipline. My Walmart loot consisted of plant-based protein powder; no more protein bars, raw eggs, hard-boiled eggs, egg white cartons, tons of colorful veggies, tofu for the allowed protein that I could consume. Fruit was limited to just two colors, namely red and blue – blueberries and strawberries. For carbs, I had to eat rice (shocking! I know). I had to give up having milk, and here I was under the impression that fat-free milk did no harm to anyone. Where would I get my calcium then?

The meal plan challenged everything I had ever known was right. I had to eat every three hours, five meals a day, and I had to drink one gallon of water. As crazy as this all sounded to me, I was so intrigued to do this, I wanted to do this, to break all norms and achieve a greater aim, to win the unknown. I also wanted to challenge my ethnicity as an Indian woman who covers herself and never should show or flaunt her body. I wanted to get completely out of my comfort zone. I had a venue to meet my abdominal muscles finally after eons and eons of challenging work.

I looked at all the food that I had purchased from Walmart; I needed to plan the weekend to do meal prep. I had to be ready for the workweek, and all the juggling to which I was accustomed. Now, in addition, I had to follow a carefully planned and measured meal plan. Initially, my first impression was that this was a lot of food!! But I was excited to take it as a challenge when the pandemic was brewing in other parts of the world.

Chapter 2: Let the fun begin.

Week one of my prep kicked off with all the excitement of a gourmet chef discovering a secret ingredient. Picture this: over the weekend, I went on a covert mission to handpick and procure the most elusive items from the wilderness caves of the grocery store. These ingredients were so exotic they practically had their own passports. As D-day arrived, my kitchen island resembled a battlefield, with rows of colorful soldiers standing ready for the culinary showdown. I even had a set of measuring cups and a food scale that looked like it belonged in a laboratory. I was a mad scientist, but instead of creating monsters, I was crafting meals that would make even Gordon Ramsay raise an eyebrow.

For my epic twenty-five-week culinary adventure, I needed a treasure trove of ingredients that could rival the inventory of a gourmet wizard's pantry. Brace yourselves, folks, because this shopping list reads like the lineup for a quirky, avant-garde food festival:

- ☐ Gluten-free oats (for that fancy touch)
- ☐ A box of strawberries and blueberries (because who needs just one berry?)
- ☐ Unsweetened almond milk (cows are so last season)
- ☐ Black beans (the dark knights of legumes)
- ☐ Organic tofu (for the health-conscious space cadets)
- ☐ Rice cakes (the unsung heroes of snack time)
- ☐ Almond butter (peanut butter's sophisticated cousin)
- ☐ Raw eggs (rock 'n' roll breakfast)
- ☐ Precooked boiled eggs (for when you are feeling extra lazy)
- ☐ Egg white cartons (because egg yolks had their moment)
- ☐ Broccoli and Spinach (for the Popeye in all of us)
- ☐ Ten pounds of jasmine rice (because we are in it for the long haul)
- ☐ Ezekiel bread (bread so righteous it has its own fan club)
- ☐ Organic plant protein powder (made from the tears of vegan unicorns)
- ☐ Green beans, zucchini, fresh greens salad, and cucumbers (the green dream team)

And that is just the beginning, folks. Stay tuned for more culinary escapades as I embark on this gastronomic odyssey! □□□

I had to follow five carefully measured balanced macro meals of Carbohydrates, fat and protein and unlimited greens added to every meal. Meal Prep Madness! Here is how I orchestrated my own culinary symphony:

Meal one:

For my breakfast masterpiece, I opted for the six-egg-white veggie omelet from the office cafeteria. Why bother making it at home when you can let the cafeteria wizards work their magic, right? Plus, it is an excellent excuse to avoid setting off the office fire alarm with my culinary skills.

Meal two:

Now, let us talk about the morning concoction that turned my kitchen into a laboratory. It all started with precisely one cup of strawberries. I am not kidding; I counted them. It took six medium-sized strawberries to fill that measuring cup. Then, I tossed in a handful of baby spinach, some unsweetened almond milk, and not one, but two scoops of plant protein. Behold, the morning smoothie of champions! I even found a snug spot for it in my lunch bag, like a proud parent sending their smoothie off to school.

Meal three:

Lunchtime, my friends, was a dazzling display of colors on my plate. I mean, it was like Picasso had a hand in crafting this masterpiece. First, I would like to give a shoutout to my pre-soaked black beans, because nobody likes a lunchtime gas explosion. Then came the tofu, about twelve medium-sized cubes of it, ready for action. I gave those little tofu soldiers a quick spray of fat-free oil, a sprinkle of salt and pepper, and threw them into the air fryer. Presto! A healthy lunch that did not just taste good but also had its own little culinary adventure story to tell.

Meal four:

Rice cakes, almond butter, and a bonus round of 25g of plant protein. I gazed into my pantry, and there they stood, the individual cartons of organic plant protein, in chocolate and vanilla flavors. No need to pack these bad boys since I would be home by then, ready to enjoy the protein party.

Meal five:

This one was all about pure protein, with a sidekick of dark veggies. And guess what? I had a secret weapon in the form of boiled eggs—pre-boiled, pre-shelled, and prepped for action and no carbs for the night a-ah! They were ready to roll, just like my determination to conquer meal prep madness!

After a rigorous and meticulous Sunday night kitchen session, I orchestrated a culinary masterpiece, carefully arranging my meal boxes in the fridge. With a satisfied kitchen cleaning session to cap it off, I knew this kitchen would see a lot more action. As the saying goes, "Abs are made in the kitchen," and my abdominal muscles were in desperate need of some TLC. The kitchen was my battleground, and it had to be in peak condition to serve my purpose. I chugged down the newly prescribed supplements, including fish oil, flaxseed oil, and multivitamins. With my project plan executed and the first sprint deliverable achieved, I crawled into bed, radiating optimism.

Lying there, gazing at the ceiling in the semi-dark room, I was brimming with enthusiasm. I was determined to eat right, get healthy, be accountable, and make a real difference. I had encountered the never-ending maze of web articles on healthy eating in the past, and they always left me baffled. To complicate matters, being a vegetarian limited my options for crafting a perfect macros-based meal.

Filled with anticipation for what tomorrow would bring and sporting high spirits, I enjoyed a restful night's sleep. The following morning, I awoke before the sun had even risen. With enthusiasm coursing through me, I swiftly packed my lunch bag, donned my gym attire, slung my gym bag with my office clothes over my shoulder, and grabbed my laptop bag. Racing down the deserted interstate, I reached the office in no time, as it was still 5:30 am, and there were hardly any signs of life on the road.

I expertly parked my car in front of the gym, moving with purpose as I entered the building. Knowing that the elevator would not be operational until 6 am, I opted for the stairs. Balancing an array of bags that made me resemble a circus act, I opened the door to the office area. At this point, I did not care how comical I looked; it had become a daily routine. I placed all my belongings at my desk, connected the laptop to its docking station, and powered it on, all in the semi-darkness of the empty floor. I quickly logged in and perused my emails, mentally charting out the day's requirements. The office floor gradually lit up at 6 am, signaling it was time for me to head downstairs. With a water bottle in one hand and my gym bag in the other, I sprinted down the stairs, finally arriving at the gym's entrance. The gym entrance door remained closed, so I patiently waited, gazing at my Member of the Year poster adorning the wall. I felt an immense sense of pride in my achievements and goals, serving as my own inspiration to continue pushing the boundaries in bodybuilding.

Finally, the coach arrived and swung open the door to the gym, which I considered a sacred temple, a Zen sanctuary where all my troubles and thoughts would be vanquished, and to finally meet my six pack abdominal muscles would be achieved. I promptly signed in at the computer and hurried to the ladies' locker room. After securing my belongings in the locker bearing my name, I could not help but revel in the fact that I had my own personalized locker for an entire year a- perk for being recognized as a member of the year, a privilege reserved for distinguished members like me. My name was boldly engraved on an image of a golden cup affixed to the locker door. With my hair tied up, hairband in place, and a confident flex of my biceps in the mirror, I flashed a winning smile at my reflection before heading into the gym to conquer the weights.

Typically, I attended classes in the morning, but due to my preparation for the competition, I had been instructed to engage in fasted cardio sessions to maximize fat burning. Research has shown that while we sleep, our bodies undergo recovery and repair, using up glycogen stores for limb recovery.

So, when engaging in steady-state cardio in the morning, the body craves energy to move, and since glycogen stores are low at that time, the body taps into its fat reserves to provide the necessary energy. This practice was crucial for my progress, and I had to make fast cardio a consistent habit in the months ahead. With my headphones on, I tuned in to my favorite music and proceeded to stretch my quads, hamstrings, and glutes before stepping onto the treadmill for a steady-state run. The group fitness room was abuzz with the morning class led by the coaches. Normally, I would have relished joining this energetic class for the camaraderie, group constructive collaboration, and invigorating workout, but now I was on a mission that demanded strict adherence.

After a satisfying workout, I headed to the showers and got dressed. Back at my desk, I stashed my sweaty gym clothes beneath it and logged back into my computer. Feeling refreshed, slightly hungry, but filled with enthusiasm, I eagerly embarked on the new week's journey. The cafeteria would open in thirty minutes, and I was ready for my first meal of the day, consisting of a six-egg white protein serving, boasting a hearty 25g of protein. As I descended the three flights of stairs to the cafeteria, my credit card in hand, the tantalizing aroma of freshly prepared food filled the air, creating an irresistible blend of scents.

I strolled over to the "Make Your Egg" kiosk, ready to place my order for a custom-made 6-egg white veggie omelet. The lady at the counter eyed me curiously and quizzically asked, "Are you sure about 6 egg whites? That's two big scoops, you know."

I confidently replied, "Absolutely, bring on the eggstravaganza!" To my amazement, she poured the egg white liquid onto the hot grill, and it started spreading like an Antarctic ice shelf. It was massive! While the eggs sizzled and transformed into a sprawling sea of white, she expertly grilled an assortment of veggies to the side. I was in for a breakfast treat fit for a monarch—well, in this case, a queen. Yes, I decided I was a queen, and it was high time I treated myself as one.

I triumphantly returned to my desk, clutching this precious loot, with the grand ambition of devouring it alongside half a cup of oats, seasoned with a dash of salt and cinnamon. Those oats had been lovingly packed in a small Tupperware container over the weekend.

But wait, before I could dive into this royal feast, I had an important task at hand. I needed to take a snapshot of my majestic meal and send it off to my coach. You see, it was a mandatory ritual for all us newcomers, lasting at least a month—capturing each meal and seeking the coach's approval. I had never been the type to photograph food; I was more of a "let's dig in" kind of person. But here I was, documenting my culinary creations for the coach's blessings. Bow to the breakfast queen!

As I diligently snapped photos of my meals, I also had a high-tech backup plan to ensure I did not forget a single bite. My phone was rigged with alerts and reminders, turning me into a mealtime ninja.

Halfway through conquering my colossal omelet, I faced a surprise breakfast intruder—Marianna, my cube neighbor. She glanced at my food mountain with raised eyebrows.

"Good morning, oh my, that omelet is bigger than a sumo wrestler's breakfast!"

"Hey, Marianna," I replied between bites, "Remember that crazy idea I had about entering a bodybuilding competition? Well, guess what? I met with the coaches last Friday, and my journey officially starts today." I could not help but whisper-squeal, trying to contain my excitement within our hushed office surroundings.

Marianna's eyes lit up with excitement. "That's amazing news!"

"But, Marianna," I said, leaning in closer and lowering my voice conspiratorially, "Let's keep this between us. I am not entirely sure if I am capable of this. What if I fail?" Marianna did not respond but her eyes did. She eyed the massive omelet, wondering if I would finish it.

Finish it I did, though not without a battle. Thanks to the veggies and jalapeños, that omelet packed a flavorful punch, and I was proud to prove that I had the appetite of a seasoned bodybuilder in training.

As I stared at the remaining half-cup of oatmeal, I could not help but feel like a contestant on a crazy breakfast game show. My stomach was sending S.O.S. signals to my brain—"Mayday! Food overload!" In a valiant effort to regain my composure, I sipped on some water and wobbled off to the restroom. Upon my return, my tummy was trying to make a subtle escape from my office pants, like a rebellious balloon slowly inflating.

But lo and behold, I was experiencing the strangest sensation. The introduction of all this protein had transformed me into a content and well-fed human being. It is like my stomach was shouting, "Hallelujah! We have sustenance!"

Marianna, being the food detective she was, could not resist inquiring about the fate of my colossal omelet. "So, did you conquer that Everest of an omelet?" she quipped.

"Oh, you bet! I even polished off half a cup of oats," I replied with a chuckle. Marianna and I have shared countless conversations about health, food, and fitness over the years. Little did I know, within the walls of our office building, there were a few undercover NPC state-level bodybuilders! These ladies were like secret fitness agents, hiding in plain sight, exuding potential, and sheer capability. These incredible women embodied true power, transcending the boundaries of their own limits, both mentally and physically, to reach their formidable goals of endurance. What struck me was that, beyond their awe-inspiring physique, these professional bodybuilders led lives just like the rest of us—filled with personal commitments, families, and work responsibilities. Their tenacity was nothing short of astonishing, a true testament to the human spirit. It ignited a fire within me, a burning desire to become one of them.

As thoughts of bodybuilding swirled in my mind, I embraced the day with a renewed sense of vigor and purpose. But it was not all smooth sailing. The task of consuming a gallon of water each day proved to be a daunting challenge. I had to remind myself constantly to take those sips. And when I did, it felt like my stomach was staging a rebellion, puffing up like a stifling air balloon. The coaches assured me it would pass, but the commitment to drinking a gallon daily remained steadfast.

In addition to the water marathon, I had to consume meals every three hours. Occasionally, I would get so engrossed in eating that I would forget the all-important task of taking a picture to send to my coaches, often capturing half-eaten dishes with a sheepish apology. In that first week, I was far from achieving the one-gallon water goal, and I could not help but wonder how the seasoned competitors managed it. To me, the idea seemed utterly insane! Yet they did it, and I was determined to learn their secret.

The solution was clear: I needed to start a conversation with these remarkable women, to reveal my aspirations and dedication to the journey ahead. As soon as the dialogue began, it was like reuniting with old friends who shared the same passion and dream. We became allies, eager to uplift and empower each other as women. It was an unspoken bond of sisterhood, and I felt honored to be part of this empowering community. Of course, I had Bony, my friend, just a text message away. I could ask her anything, and she had assured me that she would be there for me through it all. It is fascinating how a shared interest can bring people together, transcending differences in backgrounds or origins. When you discover that common ground, conversations become vibrant, two-way exchanges filled with details, enthusiasm, and vitality.

As I chatted with all these individuals who had previously competed, I soaked in a wealth of information: input, feedback, tips, tricks, advice, and recommendations that would prove invaluable on my journey. My notepad was quickly filling up with these precious insights. My adrenaline was pumping, and I was riding high on spirits, feeling like there was an entire universe of knowledge to explore within the realm of bodybuilding.

By the end of that first week, I could not help but feel a sense of accomplishment. I had successfully completed an entire week of consistent meal prep and training. My daily routine consisted of devouring generous quantities of food across five meals, and it left me feeling not just physically balanced but mentally as well. In terms of my workouts, my first week included three sessions of thirty-minute cardio in the morning and four weightlifting sessions in the evenings, thoughtfully spaced out. These weight training sessions were divided into three categories:

1. Push Muscles Workout: Here, my focus was on chest, shoulders, and biceps.
2. Pull Muscles Workout: This session was dedicated to working on my back and triceps.
3. Legs: I homed in on my quads, hamstrings, and calves, giving my lower body the attention it deserved.

Abdominal muscles: I had to do it every other day to strengthen my core had to do push one day, pull another day and two days of Leg workouts with weights in a week. The five meals a day and each meal had to comprise of 25 g of protein, seventy-five grams of carbs. Thinking of it and saying it many times was not going to get it any simpler, but I felt a sense of ownership and purpose.

As I wrapped up my first week, I could not help but feel a sense of accomplishment. I had remained steadfast in my commitment to balanced and healthy eating, and I was proud of the choices I had made with a clear goal in mind. So, on that Friday morning, I gingerly stepped onto the weight scale, half-expecting it to tell a different story. But to my utter surprise and delight, the scale revealed that I had shed 1.5 pounds in just one week of following the plan! I was genuinely impressed. It was almost magical; here I was, consuming more food, yet it was the right kind of nourishment, and I was losing weight. It made me feel not just lighter but stronger, and that was an incredibly cool sensation!

Buoyed by this optimistic and powerful positive thought, I approached the rest of my day at work with renewed energy. However, as mid-afternoon rolled around, an unexpected announcement sent everyone in my department scurrying to the big conference room downstairs. You know how impromptu meetings can either be fantastic or dreadful? Well, the urgency with which we were summoned certainly piqued my curiosity. I grabbed my trusty water bottle and strolled into the conference room, settling into a chair, and observing my colleagues trickling in, all while sipping from my water bottle because a woman's got to finish the gallon every day.

As everyone filed into the conference room, there was an unmistakable air of curiosity and anticipation. I glanced at my director, her composed demeanor suggesting that this was no harbinger of sad news we were about to receive. Once the room settled into an expectant hush, our leader took her place at the front and began by expressing gratitude for our prompt attendance, assuring us that the meeting would be brief. As her words resonated through the room, I found myself listening with a mix of personal interest and selfish enthusiasm. My director broached the subject of the Coronavirus, detailing its origins and rapid global spread. The official announcement, she conveyed, was that the World Health Organization (WHO) and the Centers for Disease Control and Prevention (CDC) had declared a pandemic. The virus was surging within the United States.

At first, I could not help but wonder what all this had to do with our daily corporate tasks. However, as the meeting unfolded, the pivotal revelation came and we were granted permission to work from home, effective immediately. It was as if the school bell had rung for a young, excited student, and I was dashing home with glee. You see, I rarely spent much time at home before. Balancing family and work throughout the years had always been a challenging yet rewarding endeavor. From dawn till dusk, I was perpetually on the move—shuttling the boys to soccer, guitar, violin, and gymnastics, and then whipping up meals for my ever-hungry clan after a demanding day at the office. My schedule left little room for respite, let alone leisurely strolls around our picturesque neighborhood to commune with the wise, old trees.

As I made my way home, thoughts of my bodybuilding competition prep swirled through my mind. Preparing meals at home would undoubtedly be more convenient, with the kitchen ready at hand. Thankfully, being a member of two gyms meant I could easily pivot to the local one near our house should I be unable to make it to the office gym. In that regard, I was all set. But then it hit me—I hoped my college-aged son would be home with us during this time. It was a realization that carried a glimmer of hope.

Upon arriving home, I logged in to work remotely and then texted my husband to fill him in on the day's unexpected turn of events. Our home, as always, was a bit of a mess. My bustling schedule had left little time for meticulous housekeeping; everything was functional but rarely in impeccable order. Little did we know that the weekend marked a turning point, not just for our family but for the entire world, as the CDC declared the onset of a pandemic. The word "pandemic" had always been foreign to me, but now its weight bore down upon my thoughts. Concern for my family's safety took center stage, and I was determined to ensure we were well-prepared as we settled into our homes, ready to play our part in saving the world. That weekend was a whirlwind of activity—grocery runs, stockpiling dry goods, and a mad scramble for toilet paper and hand sanitizers.

My older son returned home, his return reluctantly, as if torn from the midst of a crucial semester. Adjusting to home life while continuing his studies proved challenging, but he was back because his university had shut down. He looked like a disheveled mess, a common sight for him. University life had its way of wearing him down, especially since it was his first time living away from home. However, he remained an exceptional student, unwaveringly focused on his goals. I was relieved he was safely back with us, away from the looming threat of the deadly virus. Then, the news came that my husband would also be working from home and then the middle schooler son was on his way home as well. In a twist of fate, we found ourselves all under one roof. Our first order of business was to carve out designated, organized workspaces for each of us as we embraced the virtual work world.

Given the urgency of the situation, I claimed the upstairs study room as my workspace, mainly because it was the only room equipped with a speakerphone—an essential tool for my job that was now dominated by constant calls. My older son, on the other hand, had an unconventional approach. He insisted on setting up his workspace near the kitchen, believing that a bit of noise and activity helped him concentrate. It was an odd choice, considering my preference for a quiet environment, but I did not question it too much. Everyone had to adapt in their own way. My younger son retreated to his room with the shared laptop, ready to dive into his schoolwork. As for my husband, he commandeered the dining room as his remote office. Our impromptu home offices were established in haste, but we were set up and ready to tackle our work from the confines of our home.

Chapter 3: We all fall.

As we entered the era of the "new normal" (yes, that term was practically tattooed into our brains), the world outside became a source of panic. Fear clung to every human interaction, and even a mere cough or sneeze sent shivers down our spines. Suddenly, the term "corona" was no longer associated with a refreshing beverage, but with a deadly virus that was making headlines worldwide. The virus's ambiguous symptoms blurred the lines between common cold and potential death sentence, leaving us in a constant state of perplexity. The constant barrage of news only fueled our doubts, causing collective brain to drain and a sense of mind-numbing confusion. Yet, despite the uncertainty, we found solace in being together under one roof and decided to get organized.

But little did we know that what started as a family reunion would soon turn into a slow-motion comedy of errors. Life, as it often does, decided to play tricks on us. We were cut off from the outside world, life was revolving in our household with just the players of my family. We were confined and got into each other's ways like never before. Privacy was fading with the dawn of ever new day. Monotony and being cooped up at home became stifling. The news and media on the other hand, which was the only contact with the state of the end of the world was depressing.

If you are a news addict, and all you hear are the words Virus and its symptoms and in this dystopian lifestyle that we had to unexpectedly adapt to was the only way in these unusual times, the challenge of a powerful mind can go both ways to protect and to destroy. The lockdown meant no social interactions or gatherings. Yet, now, home had to accommodate our work, relaxation, and everything in between. Prolonged confinement led to strange consequences—reports of lockdown-induced depression and fatigue, illustrating the unprecedented nature of our predicament.

With a deluge of negativity, maintaining optimism and positivity became increasingly challenging. However, it was also a time to cherish the safety and well-being of our loved ones. If we followed protocols, we believed we were safe at home.

I awaited my gym sessions like a lifeline through all these changes that overcame my household, and we were singled out from the rest of the world in these unusual times. But then, disaster struck! The rumor mill churned out news that gyms were closing. Panic set in. The gym was my sanctuary, my escape from the madness of the world. It was my haven, my fortress of solitude. It was the one place where I could pretend to have it all together. I felt trapped and disheartened, drowning in despair. As I wallowed in melancholy, I started to doubt whether competing in the show was worth the struggle. The universe was telling me, "Not today, buddy." The tunnel of negativity loomed large. The lunatic in my head gleefully urged me to quit. It sang songs of despair and whispered, "This isn't meant for you." It was a relentless mental torture that threatened to shatter my resolve. But then, in a moment of desperation, I reached out to my savior: Bony.

I was not too deep into my prep journey at that point. It was best to quit now before it got even harder, I thought. But Bony's response was a lifeline in the sea of doubt. She understood my predicament, having experienced her own lockdown without gym access. She reassured me that there is never a "good time" for prep; you just must do it. That phrase echoed in my mind. The universe, it seemed, was tossing me a lifeline amidst the chaos. With renewed determination, I decided to dive headfirst into my prep. Challenges were opportunities in disguise, and I was ready to seize them.

There is always a positive aspect in every situation; we just need to adjust our perspective to embrace it and bask in its glow. Meal prep emerged as my newfound superpower, transforming my kitchen into a realm where I reigned supreme, armed with an iron skillet. Perhaps this marked the genesis of Iron Chic and the thrilling odyssey toward my NPC bodybuilding aspirations.

Having my kitchen at my disposal meant freshly cooked meals, eliminating the need for cumbersome pre-planning and reheating lunches at the office—a significant boon amid the lockdown.

Furthermore, I found myself liberated to cater to my own culinary needs, unencumbered by the expectations of others. I diligently measured every meal, scrutinizing my macros for the first time in my life. Amidst cooking for my family, I carved out precious moments to prioritize my own nutrition. The impact was palpable within weeks as I adhered to a rigorous meal plan—I shed pounds, felt a surge of strength, and, most importantly, liberated myself from the constraints of family dinner scrutiny. It was a revolution unfolding within the sanctuary of my own home.

However, the true test lay in my training regimen. How could I rise to meet it? The voice of audacity within me whispered a daring suggestion—transform my living room into a makeshift gym, where my dumbbells awaited as steadfast allies. Thus began a surreal metamorphosis, where the "new normal" transformed into a theatrical spectacle in which I played the starring role, deftly juggling responsibilities and vanquishing doubts with each rep.

Like a beacon of hope breaking through the darkest of times, I stumbled upon a treasure I had long overlooked. Tucked away amidst neglect, a set of dumbbells from COSTCO waited patiently, untouched for years. My heart soared as I realized the potential for progressive overload style weightlifting nestled within. Ranging from 10lbs to 35lbs, these dumbbells promised versatility for sculpting my body in countless ways.

With gyms shuttered, I embraced this discovery with fervor. Transforming our humble family room into my sanctuary, I repurposed a simple foldable party chair into my throne, and a folded comforter became my haven for floor exercises. Despite the absence of fancy machinery, I found solace in the simplicity of my makeshift gym.

But it didn't end there. Beyond the confines of walls, I found vast opportunities awaiting in our front and backyard. With determination as my guide, I embarked on lunges and squats upon the sturdy pavers, the rhythm of nature serving as my coach. Each rep was punctuated by the symphony of wind and birdsong, while the crisp oxygen invigorated my spirit.

In the face of adversity, I discovered not only the means to continue my journey but also the beauty of embracing nature's gym. With each lift and stride, I forged a path towards strength and resilience, finding joy in the simplicity of my surroundings and the boundless potential within myself.

Next was in the dusty garage, an eighteen-year-old bicycle and a neglected treadmill stood ready for action. In the face of adversity, I channeled my inner determination. Where there is a will, there is a way, I reminded myself. I transformed my home into a sanctuary of fitness. It was a revelation, a testament to the power of resourcefulness. With unwavering hope, I continued my training and diet regimen, setting my sights on my goals. I tuned out the negativity surrounding me and let my progress speak for itself. Home life remained challenging, the world outside grew bleaker, but the virtual realm offered solace.

I deliberately disconnected from the relentless news cycle. There was no time for it. My days were a whirlwind of responsibilities—caring for my boys, cooking, cleaning, working from home, and, of course, dedicated training and prep. I became a well-oiled machine, unfazed by the chaos the pandemic wrought upon the world. Quitting was not an option. I thrived in my newfound routine. I embraced my supermom status, adept at multitasking. My home and family had always been my training ground for juggling myriad responsibilities. Now, with a clear goal in sight, everything else paled in comparison. My determination blazed brighter than ever.

Chapter 4: The worst was yet to come.

Florida continued to sink deeper into despair as the number of cases relentlessly climbed, reaching a staggering eight thousand infected individuals. The cumulative death toll, an ever-increasing testament to the grim reality the world was facing for the very first time. The state, besieged by the unyielding virus, was forced into a grim lockdown, a final effort to halt the relentless spread.

Only essential services managed to retain a semblance of normalcy, while the rest of the world crumbled under the weight of uncertainty. The state governor wielded the iron fist of restriction, decreeing a draconian order that curtailed movements and personal interactions outside the confines of one's home for an agonizing thirty-day period. In certain desolate counties, businesses shuttered their doors, and the once-bustling roads lay barren. The hospitals, once places of healing, were now overflowing with despairing patients, and the medical personnel, stretched beyond their limits, faced an endless tide of suffering. Law enforcement roamed the deserted streets, their authority unquestioned, interrogating anyone who dared to venture out into the silent abyss. Notices, like ominous proclamations of doom, were served to businesses that dared to defy the mandate, promising legal penalties as retribution. The world outside crumbled, transforming into an unrecognizable nightmare.

In the cocoon of my household, I grappled with a maelstrom of obstacles. Doubts clawed at the edges of my mind as I juggled the weight of my goals and the ceaseless demands of additional household chores and familial responsibilities. Despite the mounting challenges, the thought of surrender never crossed my mind. Quitting was not an option. My daily routine was a grueling marathon, with mornings commencing at the ungodly hour of 4 o'clock and concluding as late as 10 o'clock in the evening. I found solace in the chaos, each day a frenetic whirlwind of activity that kept me from dwelling on the world's worsening plight.

In the dim light of dawn, a typical day began with the commencement ritual: a ritualistic ingestion of coach-prescribed supplements, a peculiar concoction of BCAAs (Branch Chain Amino Acids) with water, and a dash of jal-jeera to add an Indian flavor to it kickstarts my metabolism before sunrise and before the household awakens. Clad in my dry-fit workout attire, I embark on my fast cardio journey upon the trusty treadmill. The duration of these morning runs fluctuated, dictated by my ever-evolving progress. The rationale behind fasted cardio was twofold: it was most effective in the morning when glycogen stores, depleted overnight, forced the body to rely on fat as its primary energy source. Moreover, it was imperative to maintain a steady heart rate, optimizing fat burn and not lose muscle—a delicate balance unique to everyone.

Working out before the sun's ascent was optimal; a well-rested body and mind greeted the breaking dawn with a sense of calm and anticipation. These moments of solitude, when the world slumbered and the promise of a new day beckoned, held a certain allure. The tranquility and the prospect of new beginnings provided a flicker of hope. As the rest of my household slept, I cherished the "Me, myself, and I" time—a precious commodity in these uncertain times.

Upon completing my fasted cardio, I embarked on a deep stretch followed by a warm shower. A quick snapshot of meal one was dutifully sent to my coaches, serving as a checkpoint to confirm my adherence to the program. The day officially begins for my husband, with his own routine, while I retreated to the study room to delve into my professional responsibilities. In stark contrast, my children appeared to exist in a different time zone, rising just as I prepared a delectable, cool, and healthy organic smoothie for meal two. Amidst morning kisses, hugs, and the exchange of greetings, I ensured breakfast was served for my kids, who navigated the labyrinthine virtual realm of education. Guiding and supporting them became an essential part of my daily duties.

Meal three, or lunchtime, heralded another round of culinary endeavors. I juggled the preparation of my meals alongside those of my family. During this whirlwind, I diligently sipped water, striving to meet the elusive one-gallon-a-day water consumption goal. The extra culinary duties highlighted the stark reality of our world—a world where restaurant outings and food delivery were luxuries of the past. In these dire times, we adapted, making the most of our limited provisions.

My relentless pursuit of personal goals kept me isolated from the ever-encroaching changes in the outside world. Amid the turmoil, I ritualistically photographed each meal, offering it as a digital sacrifice before consumption—a testament to my unwavering dedication. My mom's penchant for culinary presentation rubbed off on me, igniting a newfound appreciation for the finer aspects of decorating food. Each meal transformed into a canvas, a palette of colors and textures meticulously balanced to perfection. My relationship with food evolved, unveiling a path previously uncharted.

The weight of the world bore down upon us, but my goals remained a constant, a lifeline tethering me to sanity amidst the chaos. My photo gallery and text exchanges with my coach were increasingly dominated by the monotony of five pictures a day. Those same coaches, whom I had encountered in person a mere two times before embarking on this endless journey of preparation and meal plans, had now assumed the role of my most frequent social contacts—outside of the suffocating walls of home. They offered little more than cursory acknowledgment in response to my diligently documented meals, usually manifested as a thumbs-up emoji or the occasional encouragement like:

"Good choice."

"Good job, keep it up."

If I were, for whatever reason, delayed or forgetful in transmitting my meal pictures, a terse "Meal?" text would quickly snap me back to reality. I would scramble to hastily capture a photo and dispatch it to them, desperate to atone for my minor indiscretion. The daily conversations served as a lifeline, my tenuous connection to a world beyond the confines of my immediate family. They sustained my fragile focus on these elusive goals, granting me an illusory sense of strength and health amidst the gathering gloom.

Four interminable weeks had crept by each day a relentless grind. Now, it was that dreaded time of the week again—the physical check-in. This torturous ritual entailed a thorough examination of my body fat percentage and the relentless judgment of my weight at the coach's studio. My progress, or lack thereof, was distilled into these cruel measurements, which, in turn, dictated further adjustments to my already punishing meal plan. The pantry was well-stocked, and there had been no compelling reason to venture into the treacherous outside world, locked down to halt the inexorable march of a merciless virus. I awaited this weekly expedition with feverish anticipation, convinced that my unwavering discipline and unwavering efforts had yielded progress. The weight scale at home seemed to affirm my belief, as it relentlessly ticked downward. Surely, this was proof of my relentless march toward success, I reasoned.

Still, the knowledge that my aspirations hinged on these dreaded check-ins gnawed at my sanity to do better, to be better every single day. Coach Ty, with his unwavering positivity, went about the ritualistic process of measuring my body fat percentage with clinical precision. He meticulously noted down the results, juggling numbers on a spreadsheet like an unfeeling machine. Meanwhile, my eyes wandered to the overhead television, a relentless conveyor belt of sad news. More deaths, more infections, more symptoms of the virus—its relentless march was inescapable. I took a deep breath through my mask, a mask that felt increasingly suffocating, and sighed.

"I am tired of hearing the same topic everyday" I said.

"Yeah, it is crazy out there" he responded.

Turning his attention to me with a smile he said, "Ready to discuss your progress?"

"Yes, I want to know" I said.

"Definitely good progress from where you started," the coach's words carried a modicum of assurance, but it was fleeting.

"Yes!" I tried to muster enthusiasm, clinging to the intangible signs that had accompanied my dietary shift. There was more energy, a semblance of well-being, a newfound enjoyment in workouts, even amidst the oppressive confines of lockdown. Yet, I could not shake the relentless doubt that continued to gnaw at my confidence.

"Body fat percentage has seen an incremental decrease, but most of the fat has stubbornly accumulated in the ab area," he continued, and my hope waned.

"Why is it accumulating there?" I could not help but question. The eternal battle of the abdominal muscles!

"Genetics," he explained, a verdict that was as merciless as it was disheartening. It was a cruel realization that no matter how relentless my efforts, some things were beyond my control. I knew theoretically that spot-reducing fat was impossible, a cruel irony I had grappled with my entire life.

In this relentless pursuit of my goals, I had learned that a clean and healthy diet, coupled with meticulous workouts to fortify my core, was essential for building muscle. Increased muscle led to a higher metabolism, which in turn, would chip away at the stubborn fat. But as I stood there, doubts lingered like growing shadows. "Consistency is the key," he assured me, a shard of hope in his voice. "I will make adjustments to the meal plan and send it tonight. Stick to the plan, it will work for you. Just trust the process."

As I drove home, the coach's words echoed in my mind, a desperate refrain: "Trust the process." It was easier said than done. Surrendering to the uncertainty and placing my trust in an unknown outcome felt like an insurmountable challenge. Nevertheless, I had no other choice. With renewed determination, I navigated my daily tasks, each day with a juggling act—working from home, tending to my family's needs, and adhering to the formidable dietary demands. The evening brought with it the most anticipated email. In it, I found a mixture of good and sad news. Invariably, it was best to confront the sad news first, to soften the unyielding blow that would inevitably follow. My eyes scanned the measurements in the Excel spreadsheet the coach had sent me. My body was changing, but the transformation was subtle, too subtle for anyone, including my family, to notice. Doubts once again crept in, my tireless inner critic whispered ceaselessly. As I gazed at images of bodybuilders on stage on social media, a persistent stream of questions inundated my mind. Could I truly transform so drastically in a few months, armed only with these meals and workouts? The transformations I witnessed in those photos seemed fantastical, almost surreal. The steadfast cycle of self-doubt seemed endless especially since the world was ending anyway.

"Trust the process," the coach's words reverberated like an unyielding mantra. Trust it, I must.

My morning cardio routine expanded by a mere five extra minutes; a determined progression I knew I could handle. The real surprise came in the form of adjustments to my meals. Following meal three, I was forbidden from consuming any carbs, a ruthless twist in my dietary regimen. The ten bags of rice cakes I had purchased for my favorite meal now seemed a senseless stockpile. I decided to redistribute them to other meals, a desperate attempt to adapt.

Weeks passed, and I discovered that I was working with a finite set of ingredients. My unstoppable creativity became my lifeline as I endeavored to make each meal different, to combat the boredom. The food shortage crisis, driven by supply and demand imbalances, weighed heavily on my mind. The pursuit of my goals demanded ingenuity in the kitchen, as I stretched my finite resources to their limit. Then came the inevitable news: the spread of the virus had finally led to statewide lockdowns in many regions. Florida had yet to succumb, but I knew it was only a matter of time. I will not be able to go for check-ins from now on.

Text exchanges with the coaches revealed a bleak solution: I was to send front and back pictures as virtual check-ins from now on along with my weight recorded on a scale every other week. Based on these visual cues, my coach would adjust my meal plan and training requirements. It was a bleak substitute for face-to-face interactions, yet it was the only recourse available in these trying times. The universe had indeed chosen a peculiar way to test my resolve. As the coach's words echoed in my mind—

"Trust the process"—I could not help but wonder if I had the strength to persevere through these trials.

The following morning, I woke early, determined to conquer another day in my fitness journey. I embarked on my fasted cardio, my steps echoing with determination. A deviation from my usual routine led me past a nearby playground, and there, an unexpected sight halted me in my tracks.

The playground stood empty, devoid of children's laughter in this early hour, and yet, a wicker basket sat on a park bench, an ominous omen. It overflowed with freshly made tortilla chips, radiating warmth in the gentle morning light. Beside it lay a bowl of the most irresistibly fresh avocado or guacamole dip, accompanied by slices of juicy mango and fiery jalapenos. The chips gleamed and steamed in the sun, their aroma tantalizing my senses. I hesitated, my stomach growling, my mouth watering. It was a cruel temptation, a gift from the universe, or a cruel test of my resolve. I yearned to taste its forbidden bounty but realized that I could share this unexpected find with my family.

Gathering the wicker basket, my stomach rumbled with anticipation. The hunger, the yearning for a taste of the divine, swelled within me. Just maybe, I could indulge in this small luxury before taking it home, a momentary escape from the depressing grind of my never-ending pursuit.

I took one of the tortilla chips, its lukewarm embrace tempting my senses as I dipped it into the guacamole. Just as the flavors began to dance on my tongue, an eerie noise emanated from the nearby bushes, a rustle so unsettling it felt inhuman. Panic surged through me, and in an instant, I envisioned a nightmare menagerie: a Tiger, a lion, an elephant, and an alligator lurking in the shadows.

Wide-eyed, I clutched the chips and guacamole, my heart pounding with fear. My mind raced not only to protect my newfound treasure but also to safeguard my own life. Oh, how I wished I could have savored just one bite of those chips. With the sudden pursuit of deadly creatures at my heels, my survival instinct kicked in, and I ran as fast as my legs could carry me. The intoxicating scent of the food taunted me, even in the face of danger. I should have resumed my Fitbit timer to measure the duration of my fasted cardio accurately, I thought absurdly.

But then, nothing made sense. Confusion enveloped me as I lost my balance, and the precious food scattered across the grass. I scrambled to my feet just in time, resuming my escape with newfound desperation. Yet, to my astonishment, the pursuing animals seemed more interested in the fallen feast than in me. They devoured the scattered treasure with ravenous abandon. My phone's alarm jolted me awake. It was 5:30 AM, and I sat up in bed, disoriented. It had all been a dream—a senseless, absurd dream, but one that would set the tone for a series of unsettling reveries to come. Dreams of foods I could not indulge in during my rigorous prep.

It was the first sign of my body's descent into a calorie deficit, a harsh reminder that I needed to eat more. My typical day began with the familiar routine: supplements, water bottle, workout attire, and sneakers. I hopped onto the treadmill, still amused by the illogical dream that lingered in my thoughts.

As I jogged, I could not help but analyze the bizarre dream. Why had I longed for chips and guac, foods I rarely enjoyed in reality? The dream, though absurd, revealed a mental struggle—temptation versus discipline. My dream had conjured up animals as barriers to prevent me from succumbing to forbidden cravings.

My days were increasingly packed due to isolation, with work and family demands escalating. Staying busy became my escape from dwelling on unnecessary thoughts, a shield against trouble. Work and encouraging the children to keep it strong in virtual schooling and be on top of their assignments and to do well in their exams kept me occupied. They grappled with the challenges of virtual learning, missing the camaraderie of their peers, and struggling with course content. Witnessing their adaptation to limited resources was intriguing. So far, I had managed weeks of prep, adjusting to home workouts as gyms remained closed. With newfound determination, I embraced the pandemic's challenges. What could go wrong? Lockdown was inevitable; what else could the universe throw my way?

Then, an email landed in my office inbox, a harbinger of personal upheaval. It announced an alternate work arrangement I had been selected for, a corporate responsibility to assist customers impacted by Covid. As I read the message with wide-eyed apprehension, I realized I would have to relinquish my current responsibilities and assume a role on the pandemic's front lines. Without delving into the specifics, this new task presented a daunting challenge. Despite the whirlwind of changes, I was determined to maintain focus on my bodybuilding goals. A series of unexpected events unfolded, testing my adaptability and determination.

My inbox began filling with training classes scheduled for weeks. Virtual sessions introduced me to a completely new process, rules, and regulations for my alternate work assignment. Learning became a daily grind, as I juggled rising responsibilities, family, meal preparation, and the steadfast discipline of eating every three hours. Busyness became my refuge, a defense against lockdown-induced frustration and the challenges of living with the new normal. I craved information overload to drown out the cacophony of negativity and yearnings, even letting go of thoughts and fantasies about food.

Plans had to be formulated to navigate the chaos that had engulfed my life. I reluctantly set my alarm for an unearthly 3:30 a.m., sacrificing precious sleep to accommodate the ever-expanding fasted cardio sessions that now stretched to a grueling forty minutes. The morning ritual continued with the preparation of my high-protein breakfast, followed by a busy workday that began even before my family emerged to face their own struggles.

There was no respite, no time for contemplation amidst the pandemic's pervasive gloom, the isolation of humans other than family, and the ceaseless self-doubt that gnawed at my resolve. Work had become a tenacious deity, a taskmaster that drove me through interminable days. Weeks drifted by, lost in a blur of rigorous training, note-taking, and acclimating to the demands of my newfound responsibilities. But as the weeks turned into months, time lost all meaning, descending into a nightmarish abyss of stress, tension, and eventually, despair. I found myself thrust into the frontline of my career, an unfamiliar and unsettling revelation. COVID's impact on countless Americans and their livelihoods unfolded before me, a heart-wrenching ordeal.

With each sunrise and sunset, I fielded calls upon calls, hearing tales of customers unable to pay their bills, or worse, unable to put food on their tables due to job losses during the lockdown. Empathy gradually gave way to anger and frustration, transforming my once selfless tasks into harrowing encounters with individuals pushed to the brink by the pandemic's beastly grip.

The days blurred into a depressing cycle of dealing with disgruntled customers who sought to vent their frustrations more than they sought assistance. Day by day, I served my customers during work hours, only to contend with the strains and demands of my family during the rest of my day. In the dwindling spaces of my schedule, I was compelled to adhere to my strict meal regimen. By the close of a typical day, I would muster the energy for a grueling evening of weightlifting, a form of catharsis to release the pent-up frustrations that had accumulated within me.

Working out became my refuge, a lifeline in the face of mental and physical obstacles. I refused to let my training falter, channeling my frustrations into every lift and repetition. Yet, beneath the veneer of resilience, the continuous pressures and burdens extracted their toll. I reached a breaking point, and on a fateful day, the floodgates of my emotions burst open.

I broke down, tears streaming down my face, overwhelmed by the realization that I could no longer bear the weight of my responsibilities. My mind shut down, and the cacophony of yells and the burning sensation in my chest left me gasping for breath. It was as though I was traversing a corridor with countless locked doors, oxygen depleting, engulfing me in a suffocating, gray vortex of misery.

The lockdown, the isolation, the continuous juggling of family and work, and the grueling demands of an extreme bodybuilding regimen had finally fractured my resilience. Tears flowed uncontrollably as I surrendered to the pain that had welled up within me. I had always considered myself mentally strong, disciplined, calm, and composed, thanks to my healthy lifestyle and mindfulness practices. Today, all those notions lie shattered.

Through my years of resistance training, I have cultivated a high tolerance for physical pain. My meditation practice had bestowed upon me a sense of mental balance. Yet, here I was, shattered and defeated. I ceased to care about anything; all I yearned for was an escape from the anguish that had consumed me. In an act of desperation, I composed an email to my boss, uttering the words that had become my mantra: "I want out." To my surprise, my boss responded promptly, initiating the process of relieving me from my Alternative Work assignment. I had also mustered the courage to request a couple of days off to recuperate, and that too was granted.

In those two precious days, confined to my home due to Covid, I managed to regain some semblance of sanity. I adhered to my training and meal regimen, and for the first time in weeks, I could sit in my chair and watch a movie without disturbance. Small, inconsequential things took on new value, offering a momentary respite from the storm within. Within twenty-four hours, I felt a glimmer of recovery, both mentally and physically. The human body, I realized, possessed an astonishing capacity to withstand immense pressure and tension, adapting and rebounding with resilience.

I valued my job, every breath I took, and the goals I aspired to achieve. Work still demanded an exorbitant amount of effort. The world, meanwhile, teetered on the precipice of catastrophe, with news of escalating deaths and suffering. Yet, with each sunrise, my days affirmed my newfound strength. The consistent mental torment of the past few weeks had forged a resolve within me. Clarity now prevailed in my thoughts and self-care strategies. Change had changed me; I was no longer afraid of confrontations. I had embraced change as an ally, a force that had reshaped not only my external environment but also my inner self.

I learned to divide and conquer, delegating responsibilities at home and establishing a schedule for each family member.

Chapter 5: What we think we become.

With thunder in my stomach mirroring the storm outside, I embarked on my daily training regimen in the following weeks. Even during a prolonged lockdown, my check-ins with my coaches had to be virtual. I diligently sent them my front and back pictures, allowing them to fine-tune my meal plans and workout routines. As I progressed, a transformation quietly took hold, catching me by surprise. It became evident when my clothes, once snug, began to hang loose on my changing frame.

As the external stresses of the world gradually receded into the background, I redirected my focus towards self-care and the aspirations that still beckoned. My current goal was a work in progress, a formidable endeavor that demanded unwavering dedication, time, and unwavering consistency.

My body's composition began to undergo a remarkable shift. The number on the scale slowly dwindled, a testament to my gradual weight loss. Simultaneously, my lean muscle mass surged while my body fat dwindled. This transformation painted my physique with graceful curves and newfound definition. Gone were the misconceptions that women who lifted weights would appear overly masculine; my own experience was a testament to the contrary. With each passing day, I exuded grace, my every movement underscored by the newfound muscle development that accentuated the contours of my body. Even my teenage son could not help but notice the definition in my triceps even when I was at rest. My husband, too, appreciated the positive changes, often remarking on how I radiated confidence. Encouraged by these transformations, I embraced bolder and more stylish clothing, reveling in my newfound allure and they all fit perfectly. As my physical progress became evident, my attention naturally gravitated towards food. The rumblings of hunger were now a constant companion. Food, once viewed solely as a means of sustenance, began to take on new significance.

Each week began with unwavering commitment to my fast cardio and weightlifting regimen. Yet, as the week progressed, my thoughts would invariably turn to Sunday, my weekly sanctioned cheat meal day. The value of these indulgent meals became increasingly clear. I adhered meticulously to my training schedule, dutifully following my calculated macro-nutrient meal plan, which meticulously balanced carbohydrates, proteins, and fats. With each passing day, my body entered a deeper state of caloric deficit, incinerating fat while cultivating muscle. The results were nothing short of astounding.

I navigated the week with determination, fulfilling my duties as a super mom while tending to the needs of my family and home and at this point, I was getting good at it. My forty-hour workweek, conducted from the confines of my home, propelled me forward, knowing that the weekend was drawing near - Sundays were a most welcome respite. The day would commence with an intense leg workout, a prelude to the culinary delight that lay ahead. Meal three was my highly anticipated cheat meal, a time when I allowed myself to savor the richness and indulgence, I had been denying myself. My cravings were laser-focused: pizza and dessert. I desired nothing else. These tantalizing delights awakened my taste buds, and I could hardly contain my anticipation after a strenuous workout.

One positive aspect of the COVID lockdown was the shift towards takeout and delivery from local restaurants. This transition curbed overindulgence, the temptation to dine out with friends or family, and any deviation from my training and meal plans. Cheat meals became a sacred ritual, carefully planned, and executed. I would sit down with my pizza and dessert, instructing my family to give me space and silence. With eyes closed, I would take that first bite, savoring the aroma, texture, and flavor as it danced upon my taste buds. Each mouthful was a celebration, a symphony of sensations that I cherished, bite by delectable bite. There were Sundays when I achieved the extraordinary feat of devouring an entire large pizza in one sitting, only to find myself still craving more. Reflecting on those moments now, I understand that to transform into something beyond your wildest dreams, you must be willing to tread uncharted waters.

My journey had led me down the path of a prolonged calorie deficit, reshaping my relationship with food in profound ways. At times, the hunger pangs gnawed at me, igniting a burning desire within my core that urged me to eat with an almost primal intensity. I would immerse myself in the act of eating, as if seeking redemption for the week of rigorous self-discipline. The emotional roller coaster that accompanied these cheat meals ranged from sheer delight and satisfaction to glimpses of the hardship brought about by deprivation of life's basic necessities. Tears would flow freely, celebrating the incredible flavors of something as fundamental as food. It was a poignant reminder that when you lack something, you learn to treasure it anew. I had returned to the essence of life, rediscovering the profound blessing of a world abundant with food in all its forms - a world where each color, texture, taste, and flavor told a unique story.

Amid the chaos of a rampaging pandemic, my world had shrunk to the confines of my home - my sanctuary, my workplace, my gym, my haven of Zen. I lived each day as if it were my last, savoring every moment without room for anything else. As a woman, wife, and mom, I juggled dual roles with the added responsibility of managing domestic affairs during the pandemic. I could not help but think of the countless mothers out there, mothers with young children, navigating the turbulent seas of 2020 - a year deemed a recession for women. Life was undoubtedly challenging, but after rejuvenating staycations, my thoughts turned to the immense blessings bestowed upon me.

These blessings became the bedrock of my resilience. Introspection took on a new meaning, fostering gratitude and a newfound appreciation for healthy eating habits. I realized how ungrateful I had been in the past, taking the abundance of food for granted. I had been overly particular about taste and had let preferences dictate my relationship with food. Now, I understood that the world held only a finite set of ingredients, and during my intense preparation, these options became even more restricted. I became a paragon of prudence and culinary ingenuity, delving into the realm of food inspiration. I reveled in the world of food porn, losing myself in the exquisite imagery and recipes that graced social media. It was an almost transcendent experience, akin to an orgasm of the senses. The allure of forbidden fruit fueled my creativity, leading to culinary improvisations that aligned perfectly with my macros.

For instance, I introduced a variation of French toast to my breakfast routine - a humble version that adhered to my nutritional goals. Mixing cardamom, cinnamon, and nutmeg into a cup of egg whites, I created a frothy solution. I then soaked two slices of Ezekiel Bread and toasted them in a pan. The result was a heavenly breakfast that kickstarted my day, accompanied by sugar-free, fat-free, carb-free Walden Farms syrup or jam. This journey was not just about physical transformation; it was an awakening of the senses, a celebration of gratitude, and a testament to the power of perseverance in the face of adversity.

Meal two remained a delightful cup of fresh blueberries or six succulent strawberries, accompanied by a plant protein powder smoothie, providing a refreshing and nourishing start to my day.

As I progressed to meal three, I embarked on a culinary adventure that transformed this daily ritual into a vibrant and mouthwatering experience. Utilizing the delectable Ching's spicy Schezwan sauce, I skillfully sautéed an array of colorful vegetables to perfection. To this flavorful mix, I added half a cup of wholesome brown rice and a delectable egg scramble, crafting a dish that redefined the concept of Fried rice. Each bite was a testament to my culinary prowess, and I relished every morsel with unabashed joy, savoring each spoonful down to the very last scrape from my bowl.

Meal four held a special place in my heart, resembling a dessert for the twilight hours. Rice cakes adorned with luscious almond butter, complemented by a plant protein shake, transformed this meal into a delightful treat that brought sweetness to my evenings.

While meal five ventured into the realm of zero carbs, it presented a unique challenge. Yet, I compensated by embracing a colorful array of vegetables, filling my plate with vibrant and nutrient-rich offerings. As I settled in for the night, I sought a comfortable position to sleep, determined to withstand the occasional pangs of hunger brought on by the absence of carbohydrates.

On the surface, this meal plan represented a departure from my usual dietary habits, but I quickly adapted, adhering to it with unwavering dedication. It was a testament to the incredible adaptability of the human spirit - our ability to thrive and persevere, regardless of the circumstances. Days and weeks passed, filled with rigorous training and unwavering commitment, leaving me with little time or energy to dwell on the separation imposed by lockdown.

Sugar was an entirely different realm, a realm where I found myself utterly powerless, particularly when it came to the seductive allure of dark chocolate. Its sinful, celestial darkness had long been my muse, a captivating temptation that had ensnared my senses even before my preparation journey began. Yet, the story of my relationship with sugar took on a far deeper hue after I grappled with gestational diabetes during pregnancy. In the wake of that experience, I received stern warnings from medical experts, cautioning me to tread cautiously when it came to both carbohydrates and sugar. Their concern stemmed from the knowledge that I harbored a predisposition to develop chronic diabetes.

The years that ensued were marked by a meticulously crafted, regimented, and unwavering commitment to avoid all things sugar related. I allowed myself to indulgence only on rare occasions, such as birthdays, joyous celebrations, or blissful vacations. The haunting memories of pricking my finger five times a day, the cruel routine of monitoring my blood sugar levels, continued to linger in my consciousness throughout the passing years. More than anything else, it was an ever-present fear that served as the driving force behind my determined efforts to maintain a sugar-free existence. Despite the daunting challenge of existing within a state of sugar blockade, I remained vigilant and had it all firmly under control—until the fateful day when my resolve was put to the ultimate test, being challenged, and reduced to mere dust.

True to its name, I began to dabble in the world of cheat meals, succumbing to the siren call of my all-time favorite dessert: the infamous Tiramisu. Tiramisu, a culinary masterpiece like no other, stood as a revelation and a creation that humanity had been bestowed with. If it were within my power, I would have gladly shrunken to the size of a peanut, traversing the circumference of the Tiramisu plate, indulging in its monumental Sucrose-laden delights until the world around me spun with delightful dizziness.

The darkness of the espresso chocolate enveloped me like a velvety abyss, its rich texture reminiscent of a lady's delicate finger tracing over my senses. The crème, with its silky embrace, caressed my palate, and it was all about the sensations that unfurled. Indeed, with sugar, it transcended the mere act of consumption. Rather, it was akin to descending in slow motion, falling gracefully into the heart of a decadent cake. Dark chocolate shavings encircled me like a warm embrace, and I sank leisurely into the sands of pristine white crème, allowing it to consume me entirely. Such is my indulgent vanity. If there exists one action in this world for which I bear no guilt and would readily commit to, regardless of the consequences that may follow, it is reveling in the sinful delight of this meticulously crafted, crème-filled masterpiece of human creation.

Every action carries its own set of consequences; it shapes us, molds us into what we become. Our thoughts, our choices, the nourishment we bestow upon our bodies—they all contribute to the output that our bodies reflect. The term "cheat meal," as the name implies, suggests an indulgence, an exception permitted during the grueling preparation. Yet, despite the necessity of these sanctioned transgressions, I still harbored personal doubts. I questioned my ability to transform into a figure resembling the chiseled and graceful bodybuilders I had so often witnessed on social media. In my world, it seemed as far-fetched as a scene from science fiction. Nevertheless, I was willing to embark on this journey, fully aware of the challenges that lay ahead.

The progress I observed was slow, almost imperceptible. It led me to realize the importance of patience in turning science fiction into science fact—a revelation that would become particularly evident during peak week. Clean eating, adhering to my macros, and fueling my body at regular intervals had forged me into a formidable and resilient warrior.

Cravings gripped me, akin to a pregnancy yearning. I yearned for the sweetness of sucrose, for foods that were counterproductive during this rigorous preparation. Forbidden desires swirled within me. I understood that cravings were fleeting sensations, impermanent in their nature, and needed to be kept in check. My daily meditation, lasting over an hour, became a crucial anchor, steadying my mental state. At times, it offered solace; at others, it was insufficient. As my daily cardio extended to forty-five minutes, and the intensity of my training surged, my caloric balance teetered precariously.

Chapter 6: Lockdown effects.

Evolution continued in my household and weeks went by with the intensity of a tornado. The outside evolution was also taking place with COVID testing site. Testing was rarer than a unicorn doing stand-up comedy, and they were as crowded as a clown car at a circus convention. The medical world was in an incubation period of its own, trying to figure out how to handle the pandemic-induced paranoia. News was filled with suicides of hypochondriacs due to lockdown effects.

The information about the symptoms was so vague that it had people lining up for testing like it was Black Friday at a discount store. Hospitals were packed tighter than a clown car, and they were running out of beds faster than a squirrel on a caffeine high. Those who wanted to be tested for covid received specific instructions when they arrived at the testing center: stay in the car, do not make eye or body contact with anyone, and wait for the hazmat-clad, masked, and wiser personnel to check his name. It is like they were auditioning for a role in a sci-fi movie.

The cars moved at the speed of molasses based on a first-come-first-served priority system. The hypochondriacs could only park and enter the testing room when the masked crusader told them it was their turn. An hour went by for them with stress, thoughts, and money to get tested. People were going through these strange experiences while I was busy chugging into my meals wishing the world much luck in their lives. Become a mad person in isolation or wait in never ending car lines contemplating whether you can survive on windshield wiper fluid to be tested for covid symptoms or make a difference working with the gift of time to progress your self-care or achieve a goal. It was in each one of us to make these choices during these trying times.

Isolation had driven many people to the brink, and we had all seen the news stories about it. If it were not for my strict bodybuilding regimen, I might have turned into a mad person long ago. It is true, what they say - your mind can make you a superhero or a supervillain, and in these times, we were all just trying to survive.

We were all connected virtually, depending on the power of the web and electricity to get through the day. Virtual meetings on Webex and Zoom had become the new normal, and we even got a peek into people's homes, complete with surprise appearances by pets and kids. Humor became our lifeline as we navigated this brave new world of virtual togetherness.

Social media was blowing up with activities, pictures, and videos of how humanity was adapting to the "new normal." It is like we all suddenly got on a crash course in sharing our experiences with the world. At home, we became DIY experts, attempting everything from gourmet cooking to extreme tidying-up. As my household became a Zen paradise with no emotional tension or stress, I thought, "Why not conquer social media next?"

As my abdominal muscles transformed from flabby acquaintances to taut friends, it was like I had won the lottery (a six-pack lottery, that is). And hey, when you are on the road to success, you cannot just keep it to yourself. So, naturally, I started posting videos of my creative workouts and pictures of my ever-improving physique on social media.

It became an "all about me" show, but hey, who could blame me? I was slaying in every way for this transformation. Self-love was just part of the prep process, right?

The number of selfies I took became directly proportional to the tautness of my six-pack abdominal muscles. I was bursting with excitement and had to share my journey with the world.

Social media was like my virtual gym friend, a place where I could share my fitness passion with like-minded individuals.

The feedback started rolling in, and boy, did it feel good. People were all, "Look at you, you've changed!" My posts garnered likes and comments praising my fitness prowess. I had a growing legion of followers who were inspired and empowered by my posts, and that gave me the fuel to keep going on my ponderous prep journey.

Sure, I was physically drained, sleeping like a hibernating bear, and dragging myself around due to a prolonged calorie deficit, but I was ecstatic. Hunger became my new BFF. I was downing 125g of protein, 100g of carbs, and the tiniest bit of fat, and guess what? I was hungry all the time. But who needs food when you are on the road to becoming the next superhero, right?

As the state prepared to reopen from lockdown, people were glued to the news, but I had more pressing matters on my mind - like browsing the internet for food porn. I was running a culinary fantasy league in my head. Dream dinners? More like dream disappointments! I could not eat half the stuff I was ogling. I knew some foods were like little gremlins for my body, wreaking havoc from the inside, but the heart (and stomach) wants what it wants.

Desperate to silence the rumbling rebellion in my belly, I introduced black coffee into my life. At first, I wondered how something that smelled like heaven could taste like burnt regret, but then I realized I had been missing this bitter bliss my whole life. Coffee and caffeine were my newfound allies in the battle of the bulge. It is amazing how quickly we humans adapt to whatever life throws at us. We are like cockroaches with better fashion sense – we just keep on thriving. My taste buds had gone from party animals to fussy eaters, and my sense of smell was on steroids, like I was some kind of gourmet bloodhound.

Then, the restaurants had the audacity to offer delivery options. Every time that glorious food arrived at my doorstep for my family, I could practically smell it from the next zip code. I could imagine the textures, the flavors, the ingredients dancing together in a tantalizing culinary ballet – and I could not eat any of it. It was like a food tease of epic proportions. I could have a meal with my mind and be satisfied. It was insane – not only was my body transforming, but my mind was doing somersaults too.

Chapter 7: Hope mends and then bends.

Over the course of seven weeks, a remarkable transformation took place. What initially seemed like a drastic change, shifting to remote work, soon began to feel like a confining prison when the lockdown descended upon us, locking us away from the world's embrace within the safety of our homes. Yet, amidst this isolation, I found a wellspring of creativity within me. I adapted my workouts with the limited resources available at home, but deep down, I knew that to compete at my best, I would need more advanced equipment to push my training to new heights and achieve remarkable results.

Simultaneously, my husband's too had undeniable longing for the gym. Our muscles, it seemed, had developed a memory of their own, and they were getting restless without regular workouts. Then came the hopeful news from the Governor – a glimmer of light in the tunnel. The state was preparing to partially reopen, which meant more stores would unlock their doors, and the first place on our list was a store specializing in gym equipment.

My husband did not waste a moment when he spotted a sale for a Smith Machine and a bench. It was a sign of better days ahead, a symbol of our collective resilience, and a promise that the world was gradually returning to its vibrant, bustling self. The future held the hope of rekindling our fitness journey, together, with newfound dedication and an unwavering commitment to our well-being.

With unwavering determination, my husband took a day off from his home office duties, armed himself with a mask and gloves, and arranged for a curbside pickup of a Smith Machine and bench. He delved into the depths of the internet, tirelessly scouring various websites to secure Olympic-standard barbells and plates. His dedication knew no bounds, and he spent an entire day setting up the Smith Machine right in our Master Bedroom. It was like a beacon of hope during uncertainty, and I could not have been more grateful for his unwavering support. My knight in shining armor had made a strong comeback.

He transformed into my ultimate pillar of support. The yearning for the gym was an ache I thought only time could heal, but my husband's actions spoke louder than any words. He brought the gym to our home, a gesture that warmed my heart. I could not help but wonder, where would I be without him?

Best of all, we began working out together in the evenings, inspiring and motivating each other to reach new heights with our shiny new toy that now adorned our bedroom. The sight of the barbells and plates was pure joy to my fitness-hungry soul. I introduced compound workouts like deadlifts, squats, and bench pressing, all while experimenting with isolation exercises using the cable and pulley system contraptions on the Smith Machine.

The state began to slowly reopen, and this included the studio where my bodybuilding coaches worked. I was overjoyed at the prospect of leaving the confines of home to visit them in person. Meeting my coaches and fellow fitness enthusiasts became an exciting prospect, even with the new safety norms in place. Masks and social distancing were now part of the routine, but these precautions were a small price to pay for the opportunity to interact with the world again. My enthusiasm remained undiminished.

As I entered the studio, the sounds of music, laughter, and chatter washed over me. Trivial things like this had taken on a new significance in my life, and I found myself cherishing every moment. Meeting other people, especially my smiling and supportive coaches, was an invigorating experience. My check-in was successfully completed, and as I drove home, thoughts of my measurements filled my mind. The more I shrank according to the caliper measurements, the lower my body fat percentage and the higher my muscle mass.

Reflecting on the journey so far, I realized that despite the obstacles and uncertainties of 2020, I had made tremendous progress. I had established a home gym, attended to my family's needs, balanced work, and preparation, and meticulously adhered to my meal plan. Hope had illuminated my path, guiding me through the challenges, and the future brimmed with the promise of continued growth and achievement. Hope was like a vibrant melody filling my heart, positivity surged through my veins, and anticipation for the future's stage experience had me on the edge of my seat. I could not contain my excitement as I eagerly waited for the night when my coach would unveil the much-anticipated meal adjustments.

Meeting the coaches in person to discuss my tangible progress after the weeks of lockdown added a thrilling dose of reality to my journey. Each passing day brimmed with newfound mental fortitude, even though my body sometimes felt like it had been through a war zone. In between the grind, I seized moments to hop into my car, embarking on aimless sun-soaked drives along the freeway, music blaring, simply letting go. Life was a thrilling adventure once more, and my mind was on a mission, while my body was undergoing a remarkable transformation.

Milestones were flying by, especially as my six-pack abdominal muscles became more defined, and I adopted a rakish and sinewy personality. Doubts about my transformation began to dissipate into the ether. My once-diffident demeanor was breaking through with the sheer number of selfies I took, posting them on social media, and sharing them eagerly.

Cheat meals became my cherished weekly goal, a reward for my religious dedication. I indulged as if I were during a famine, devouring desserts, pizza, and sweet treats to bolster my spirits for the coming week's challenges. It was like a scientific dance with my body, a calculated trick to keep my metabolism engaged, burning calories and fat with each cheat meal. I even ventured into last year's Halloween candy stash; nothing was safe from my bottomless hunger. I was a well-oiled machine, tirelessly pushing my limits.

Weekends became my sanctuary for rest, my sleep schedule cranked up several notches. I would hibernate, sleeping well for ten to twelve hours straight. It got to the point where my husband would cautiously peek into the bedroom to make sure I was still among the living. My sleep patterns underwent a transformation; by 7 PM, I was ready to crash, unfazed by the bustling sounds of family life in the evening. Those weeks brought me the best sleep I had ever had.

The more I delved into my training, the more I pushed myself in my workouts, the more astounding the transformation results became. My husband began to see me as curvy and seductive, especially in the clothes I had bought with the goal of fitting into them one day. Short, revealing outfits clung to my body as if they had been tailor-made for me. Everything I wore accentuated my shoulders, lats, triceps, biceps, hammies, quads, and, oh my, my glutes were getting tighter, rounder, and perkier with every passing day. Life was becoming a thrilling adventure of self-discovery, and I was loving every moment of it.

That is when I felt ready to slip into a sleek two-piece bathing suit. The outcome was nothing short of spectacular—I looked fantastic, and I could not help but be electrified by my own reflection!

My social media posts were flooded with selfies highlighting my transforming physique, and the fitness community could not get enough of it. I felt empowered knowing that I was inspiring those in the fitness industry. It was a liberating sensation, breaking free from the constraints of my traditionally conservative Indian upbringing. Many deeply ingrained notions and rules were being challenged. In a culture where Indian women are expected to cover up, I was venturing into uncharted territory, contrary to the Bollywood actors who had famously shattered those norms, gaining fame and respect for their boldness in showing skin.

Posting actively on social media about my transformation was considered culturally taboo, a potential sin. Engaging in bodybuilding, especially as a woman, was seen as a path that would inevitably lead to objectification and doubts about my character. Connecting with fellow Indians and sharing my progress felt like a forbidden act, and there was a real fear that my posts might be shared, mocked, and discussed, as if I no longer valued Indian culture.

I was raised with the belief that progress should be covert, a silent and determined journey. Success would eventually speak for itself, loudly and unapologetically. But bodybuilding shattered all those preconceived notions. My focus shifted entirely to the physical body—each change, curve, and muscle group was given paramount importance. I poured love and hard work into every individual muscle, meticulously scrutinizing and reviewing progress during check-ins. The results were physical, not mental. Success was measured by the transformation of my physique, not by the noise I made but by my unwavering dedication.

With this change in basic assumptions came a newfound boldness. I felt free to remove my shirt, proudly displaying the sinews and vascularity that were the fruits of my disciplined training. There was a sense of liberation in highlighting the challenging work I had put into sculpting my body.

I was transforming mentally and did not realize that the world and the people I care, and love were not in tandem with the change. Particularly my best friend in India, whom I thought was always my best friend and there was nothing that I could not keep from her. My pictures were shared with her from time to time, without thinking, without wondering what she was thinking about them, whether it was either pride or prejudice. She was my childhood friend; I thought it would be pride of her bestie's resolve and fortitude to take up the most challenging goal that would change her life forever. That was my pondering, not being sexualized which hurt me as if I were run over by a bus. Women are never considered and respected well, at least Indian women, no matter where they are, what they do, which year they live in or which country they belong to.

What happened? It was a regular Sunday, and I called my bestie to talk to her and to get her feedback on my transformation which blew out of emotional proportion. I thought the pictures that I had shared with her following this call I thought was well received and my friend was proud of me.

I did not realize that it would come back and bite me hard. I had committed a crime of have abused my body in my friend's eyes. I had disrespected the culture in which I was raised.

My bestie reminded me of that harsh reality in that phone call that day. Instead of focusing on the progress, the challenging work that I had embarked on with my fitness journey, the focus was on how I have flaunted my body with this goal. All she said was do not post all these selfies and videos on social media. She said she could see the progress that I was making but on the same note she said I need to be secretive about it. The whole point was lost here, for the very first time I could not agree completely with my best friend. I could not see at all, because the more I heard her talk to me this way, the more the tears welled in my eyes and started flowing.

The hardships, the nights where I had to sleep with an empty stomach, the control I had to practice or let go when my family would feast on meals that I was not allowed to have, all was reduced to vapor. Body building was a metaphor that grew to the masses in popularity. Emerged the inevitable mutations from the original meaning of the sport and I was harshly reminded that I am a woman, and my place is not in this sport. The sport becomes distorted but some of the most powerful implications that made the sport were lost because it was twisted into various interpretations that were unrecognizable to me. False impressions still existed.

Initially I tried to defend my stance, tried to seek justice for my actions, but was in vain. What is particularly interesting is how these fallacies resurge periodically with renewed fervor. I was stuck in a vicious cycle because I had to explain my original purpose repeatedly. Why did she not understand that? Was it lockdown fatigue? Had she become critical because of that and could not see the reason? If a man would do this, there would not be such criticism; I was reminded where a woman's place is to be. I could not take it no more; I told her that and hung up because I needed both my hands to support my face and the tears that flowed with intensity. I cried, wept, and with this came all the frustrations, all the challenges that I have faced so far and broke down until I was parching thirsty. It was the pandemic, lockdown fatigue, lack of carbs, chronic calorie deficit, challenges of the prep or an amalgamation of them together, I had reached the lowest level to feeling reduced to nothing, confidence shattered, lost at that very moment.

I felt crucified, I had caused this to happen, I blamed it on my actions that I changed the behavior of my bestie, I was the cause for this conflicting conversation with my bestie, but I couldn't face it anymore, she was my best friend, my everything so far, and I did not have her support this time when I needed it the most.

Reacting to all the thoughts and the emotions that overpowered me, I texted her saying "I am sorry, I cannot stop now, I have to keep going, I cannot get distracted now, I have to keep going, I will contact you only after the competition." I needed her in my life, but not now that much I knew. My husband came into the room and saw me crying. He was stumped as to why and I explained to him what had happened.

My husband my hero, be blessed for pacifying me and getting me back to a state of normalcy. What would I do without him truly? What he said was exactly what I needed to hear and accept. WE: my husband and I grew up in India; we spent our childhood in India, so our cultural background was limited to that. On the same note, all our waking adulthood we spent in the Americas so our cultural background cannot be Indian as an adult. Our mindset, beliefs, focus is more American all though we look like Indians and to a certain extent we are still Indians in nature. Twenty something years that we have spent our lives here away from India, with our trials and tribulations and knowledge is pertinent to being "American." In that same period my best friend has lived her life in India with their set of experiences that will be "Indian." There is nobody that is right or wrong here, but it is a cultural clash based on the cultural aspects and differences.

I had not thought about it the way my husband explained to me. This epiphany dawned on me that very moment. I could not find any loopholes or even argue with what he said to me. My husband's words calmed the storm immediately. It made a lot of sense. Through the years of living in this country of accepting, adjusting, and adapting have changed us for the better. Usually, I have heard stories of the first generation Indian born American kids who have clashes based on the name of culture living in America. There is even a popular term for it, ABCD (American born confused Desi). My husband and I were Desi's, but we had become Americans. Like any average American, we respected the sport of body building and not sexualized it. The mindset had changed dramatically, and it was not an overnight change, but a gradual change of acclimatizing to this beautiful county we made as our home. In this situation we the immigrants were the confused desis or at least I was until this enlightenment, not the first generation: my boys.

Now all I had to do was to wipe my tears, keep my chest up, chin up and smile. I knew I had heedlessly wasted a lot of calories crying, I had lost water, so I had to replenish periodically, and my prep had to continue.

When my hope was lowest, my husband was a ray of sun that escaped through a rent in the cloud. I had an arduous and challenging task ahead of me.

My foreboding abated and going on from here was the bravest thing I ever did, without my bestie's support. I was growing up, doing things that I never thought I would, reminding that I was not going back, sideways but straight ahead with Project: Self-care and development with a weird sense of liberation.

The result was amazing, I was my own person, I had ideas of my own, and this was a turning point in the way I started thinking: Independently. With resolve and fortitude and trusting in providence, I got up and seized the day, I had so much work to do.

Chapter 8: To Flaunt or not to Flaunt that is the question.

"If you've got it, flaunt it!" This became my mantra as I boldly broke free from the shackles, the bonds, and the dogmas that had been ingrained in me since childhood. I was a fearless warrior stepping out of my comfort zone, ready to unlock a world of new experiences within the realm of bodybuilding. My first challenge: learning how to pose.

Posing in class was an unforgettable experience. On a vibrant Saturday, I drove up to the studio to attend the beginner's posing class. The studio was my sanctuary—a place where I could meet my coaches, be surrounded by those who revered the sport, and where judgment had no place. The studio was alive with activity, exuding warmth, and camaraderie. It was a place where progress was tangible and celebrated. Yes, I had to be cautious and wear a mask, but at least I had the chance to escape the confines of home, interact with fellow human beings, and dive headfirst into this new adventure.

As I entered the group room, I could not help but notice that I was obvious. I was dressed in what I considered the shortest of shorts and a tank top, while the other women sported either two-piece bikinis or shorts and sports bras, confidently highlighting their midsections. These women were living sculptures, their bodies a testament to dedication and hard work. It took conscious effort to keep my eyes from gawking; they were everywhere, reflected in the room's mirrors. I felt overdressed, bashful, and utterly out of place.

Our first task was to don heels and line up. Those heels, though they exuded sassiness, were my personal nemesis. I had never worn heels during my formative years, primarily because I had no idea how to walk in them. My attempts were comical; I was clumsy, uncoordinated, and perpetually off-balance. Plus, they made my back ache. I often wondered how women managed to walk in those contraptions. But now, I had to make peace with heeled shoes. These were not your everyday Macy's or Dillard's dress shoes; they were clear bodybuilding competition heels, towering at a daunting 4.5 inches. I had received these special heels from Amazon just a week ago, and the mere sight of them had given me the shivers. It was a hilarious spectacle as I strapped them on and attempted to walk around the house in them. The question persisted: Why on earth would anyone subject themselves to this torture?

In the opulent, marble-floored hallway that stretched for what felt like an eternity, I devoted a solid 20 to 30 minutes of my precious time perfecting the art of walking in heels. This corridor was my personal runway, and I treated it as such. In the beginning, I clung to the walls for dear life, fearing I might lose my balance—a fate that beckoned me all too often. The last thing I wanted was to suffer an ankle or knee injury. It was an unexpected twist in my journey; I had never been afraid to conquer heavy weights, push my limits, or achieve personal records in the gym. But here I was, paralyzed with fear by what seemed like a pair of Cinderella glass slippers. I just could not grasp it—I could not walk.

My gaze remained firmly planted on the floor beneath me as I shuffled along. This posture caused my back to hunch, my knees to cave inward, and my stride to resemble that of a duck. As if that were not enough, there was a significant gap between my toes and the sole of the shoe, making it impossible for them to work in harmony. With my bent back, awkwardly bent knees, and confusion over whether to step on my heels or my toes, I ended up flailing my hands on either side in a desperate attempt to maintain my center of balance. Admittedly, I must have looked fascinating with those added 4.5 inches, which made me appear taller, leaner, and slenderer. My glutes tightened, giving them a perky lift, while my calves were pushed to the limit, highlighting their newfound muscle definition. If only the stage experience involved standing still like a mannequin or adopting an akimbo stance, rather than the daunting task of walking and posing!

These heels were, without a doubt, my arch-nemesis, yet they provided endless entertainment for my family. Living in a household dominated by men had always been an adventure, and now they all clamored to try on these heels for a taste of heightened stature. It was all wholesome fun; they took turns strutting and stumbling around in their heels. By day's end, I found myself showered with empathy and support from my family as I continued to stumble and teeter while mastering this confounding footwear.

I meticulously tightened the ankle straps and, with arms outstretched to maintain balance, joined the ranks of other women who had also bravely embraced these Cinderella slippers as a necessary extension of themselves. Our first posing class proved to be a revelation. We were taught the intricate art of transitioning from our initial pose to the side, executing a flawless back pose, and then seamlessly transitioning back to the front. My performance was nothing short of a spectacular disaster. I was promptly removed from the line and assigned to receive a one-on-one lesson for dummies, an indication of just how much I needed to catch up. Posing, as I would soon discover, held immense significance in the competition. It had the power to accentuate the various muscle groups the judges scrutinized on stage.

The bikini division's poses were not merely about flaunting the body in a flirtatious and seductive manner; there was a science to it, a meticulous art form that I was beginning to unravel. This revelation transformed my perspective on posing from a chore to a crucial component of my journey.

As a certified Strong nation instructor and armed with eons of classical dance experience, there was hardly a movement I could not follow or mimic. But then came posing—a challenge unlike any I had encountered before. It might have appeared smooth and fluid when other women gracefully executed their routines, but beneath the surface lay a tangled web of intricate details I had yet to unravel. I was initially flummoxed, my footwork resembled a perplexed chicken, and I exuded all the confidence of a startled squirrel. To make matters worse, my heels and the mask concealing half my face did not exactly scream "graceful elegance."

Sensing my struggles with the heels, the coach mercifully granted me permission to shed those torturous contraptions and learn the moves barefoot. Oh, the sweet relief! With both feet back on solid ground, I rediscovered my balance and bade farewell to my aching soles. The fresh air felt invigorating, and I could finally concentrate on the nuances of the mysterious art of posing. After a series of failed attempts that may or may not have resembled interpretive dance gone awry, I began to grasp the intricacies of this complex routine. Thankfully, I was allowed to videotape the entire class, ensuring I could replay my comedic attempts at mastering the craft many times over until I got it right.

When the assistant coach felt I had reached a level of semi-competence, she led me to the group room where all the ladies effortlessly practiced their poses. Standing among them was nothing short of intimidating—they looked like goddesses who had descended from Mount Olympus, each possessing celestial bodies that defied earthly limitations. These women exuded ease and confidence with their physical personalities, while I felt like a bumbling amateur who had accidentally crashed their divine gathering.

I obediently lined up with the ladies and tuned in as Coach Jo disclosed information about the stage dynamics and how the competition unfolded. The bikini competition kicked off with group posing, followed by individual posing. Posing, it seemed, was as unique as each woman's body, tailored to accentuate our individual strengths. At least for now, I was exempt from the heels, which I promptly stashed away in their designated sack. Deep down, I knew that sooner rather than later, I would have to master those darn things.

As we commenced the group routine, I could not help but feel like an uncoordinated klutz amidst a sea of graceful dancers. I hoped beyond hope that I was blending in seamlessly, my shortcomings cleverly concealed from prying eyes. Next on the agenda was positioning in an orderly fashion at the back of the stage, following a diagonal line marked by a strip of blue tape. Even in this static stance, we were expected to strike a pose, as judges had a habit of casting their discerning gazes our way at any given moment.

And then, the moment of reckoning arrived—it was time for my individual routine. Suddenly, my mind drew a complete blank. I blurted out my confusion, desperately seeking guidance.

"How do I get to the center? Just walk?" I inquired my nerves palpable.

"Yes," came the coach's reply, delivered with an air of nonchalance. "Walk like you own the stage."

Uncertainty swirled in my mind as I approached the stage, unsure if there were any unspoken rules I might inadvertently break. My heart raced, wondering what the women before me that had done had slipped my memory. With each step, I moved forward, in a slow-motion trance, performing my front, side, and back poses before transitioning back to the front. I could not help but feel like a kindergartner emerging into the open, my cheeks flushed with shyness behind my mask. But then, something magical happened. The entire room erupted in cheers and applause. It was as if I had just taken my first steps into a whole new world.

Overwhelmed with a mix of emotions, I returned to my place in the line, sporting an enormous grin beneath my mask. My coaches offered their constructive feedback, reassuring me that with practice, these poses would soon become second nature. The enthusiastic response from the crowd boosted my confidence, gradually erasing the discomfort of venturing so far from my comfort zone. I was exhilarated, and I could not wait to share this extraordinary experience with someone who understood it all.

Before heading home, I texted my friend Bony, eager to pour out every detail of my first posting class and equally excited to hear her thoughts and advice. Our friendship had its roots in our shared fitness journeys, and she had been my initial inspiration to embark on this bodybuilding adventure. Having a friend who could relate to every aspect of my journey, someone with whom I could speak candidly, share openly, and empower mutually, was an incredible blessing. Our bond grew stronger with each passing day.

Returning home, I felt invigorated and renewed. I relived the moments, the lessons learned, and shared the video I had recorded with my family. After a quick shower, given the ongoing coronavirus pandemic with the need to not touch your face or the risks of infection spreads, I tackled the rest of the day with a newfound energy, eagerly anticipating the future and keeping my goals clearly in sight.

My admiration for the physical body that had been bestowed upon me reached new heights. From that point onward, my focus shifted, and I began to see my reflection in a different light. No longer was it about my beautiful face or perfectly styled hair; it was all about the body—its contours, curves, musculature, and vasculature. Posing became an integral part of my daily routine. I watched that videotape of my first class repeatedly, diligently practicing in front of mirrors or any reflective surface I could find. My mission: to master the art of posing and highlight the results of my hard work on my triceps, glutes, hamstrings, and that elusive slim waistline. It was a learning experience like no other, and I embraced it with open arms.

The more I delved into the world of posing, the more I realized that it was not about seduction or having any ulterior motives. It was an integral part of the bodybuilding sport—a means to highlight the ancient, strenuous benefits that come together with weight training. As I embarked on my journey, the transformation of torching fat and building muscle during my prep took on a sacred quality, akin to a religious practice. I understood that outsiders might not perceive bodybuilders, especially female ones, in this light.

My camera roll started to fill with countless pictures tracking my progress. Selfies became my way of visually documenting my journey, and every small step forward was an urge to share with like-minded individuals who cherished fitness as I did. It was a defiance of everything I had been raised with as an Indian—an act of rebellion against the cultural norms that dictated restraint, modesty, and the avoidance of any public display of one's physical attributes. Yet, I took immense pleasure in this revolutionary act, redefining my own boundaries and paying homage to the dedication, pain, sweat, and challenging work that bodybuilders invested in to achieve their goals. When you work diligently, you naturally want to flaunt your achievements.

Paradoxically, every post I made about my progress garnered an outpouring of positive comments on social media, even from people I had never met. It was as if a virtual support system had rallied around me:

"You are an inspiration."

"You've put in so much hard work, and it shows."

"What a journey! You're going to shine."

"Your transformation is incredible."

"Love your dedication. You look strong and beautiful."

"I've been following your posts, and your commitment is inspiring."

"You're absolutely kickass."

"I hope to lose weight just by looking at your posts."

These affirmations filled me with optimism, nurturing a positive mindset that radiated from within. My aura became magnetic, and the repercussions of my actions led me down a path of unbridled enthusiasm. I could not help but ponder why my best friend had reacted the way she did, all while thinking of countless women in India who remained oppressed, shouldering the burden of selfless service to humankind. For generations, they had been taught never to express their strengths, constrained by societal pressures that dictated their roles and stifled their potential.

My heart aches when I reflect upon it. It is a starkly divided world, one that lies ten thousand miles away on the opposite side of the globe, a world where enduring social stigmas persist even today.

In that world, there is a home, much like mine, and a girl like me. She is brought up with love and discipline, with the understanding that her place within the family is temporary. She is not truly considered part of the family because, one day, she will depart for her husband's house. This is the overarching goal, the very purpose of her existence. From an early age, she is trained to cook, clean, adapt, compromise, and practice selflessness. She must embrace the notion of placing her own needs above all others' and serving and loving unconditionally.

Her body must remain veiled, her demeanor conservative, her thoughts and actions conforming to a set of unwavering norms. Everywhere she goes and in everything she does, she is taught to heed the Imposter Syndrome that has been ingrained in her since birth, all because she was born a woman in a male-dominated world. Acceptance and gratitude for gender discrimination and the prevailing inequalities between women and men are instilled within her.

This way of life has been passed down through generations, evolving into new, distorted forms. Disobeying the Imposter Syndrome carries the threat of punishment, designed to instill fear within womankind. When fear alone does not suffice, mental or physical abuse at the hands of MANkind becomes their destiny.

I often find myself in deep contemplation, realizing that I am not so different from those women. The Imposter Syndrome courses through my veins, an indelible part of my being. I oscillate back and forth, replaying what transpired during that phone call with my best friend. It sends me on a roller coaster ride of emotions, stirring feelings of inadequacy and chronic self-doubt regarding actions that run contrary to the unspoken rules of accepted behavior within a group or society.

The values and roots deeply embedded in me gain strength over time, engaging in invisible battles with the new, bolder, braver, and fearless version of myself. Who is right, and who is wrong in this complex dance of values and identities? History is replete with stories of powerful women from around the globe who made a significant impact. We admire and appreciate the famous icons who initiated the feminist movement—trailblazers and activists.

Was it wrong for my friend to reiterate the values instilled in her, the values with which she was raised? Was it wrong for me not to recognize this and instead feel guilty for my actions as a bodybuilder, unapologetically highlighting every part of my body with nothing to hide?

I found myself grappling with countless questions on this matter and related topics. I was, and always will be, reminded of my Indian heritage while living the life of an American. My husband was spot-on when he remarked that our childhood was in India, but our adulthood is firmly rooted in America, which we now call home. As much as my skin bears the shade of brown, I take immense pride in being an American with Indian value systems. I should consider myself a state-of-the-art, unique product, carrying the best of both worlds and cultures.

Amidst these contemplations, spirituality emerged as a refuge, guiding me back to the fundamental aspects of human behavior. We are products of our experiences, brimming with emotions. Despite our outward differences, we are fundamentally the same, with hearts that beat as one. We share the same air and tread upon this sacred ground we call Earth. In this vast cosmos, I am but a minuscule speck of life, and even amid a pandemic, my thoughts found tranquility.

Curiously, this was the year 2020 we were discussing. The world grappled with the escalating death toll due to the virus, compounded by the growing storm of racial injustice in America, sparked by isolated incidents of racial discrimination that gave rise to the Black Lives Matter movement. In the face of such monumental issues, where did my own problems stand? I was an inconsequential nobody in this expansive universe, yet I often created a universe of significance around my own experiences.

Perspective held sway over me at times, prompting me to be more practical than reactive in my thoughts. I could not afford to succumb to stress from external factors beyond my control. Stress could elevate my cortisol levels, proving detrimental to my progress in preparation. I needed to maintain my focus on my vision, striving to achieve a significant milestone I had set for myself that year, whether it was 2020 or not. In a time when disruption had become the new norm, and change, which typically occurred gradually, had abruptly halted, we, too, had to adapt.

The crucial lesson I was learning was to be prolific rather than fixate on perfection. Our bodies and minds require reevaluation and a revisit to unleash the perfect storm of change, harnessing human traits like creativity, imagination, intuition, and ethics. The overarching question at the macro level was this: was I driving change, or was I merely being driven by it? In a world where victories and defeats unfolded at an unprecedented pace, I felt like a crucial point within the tempestuous tornado of change.

As a tiny speck of dust in this vast universe, my decision and strategy were simple: Instead of enduring constant anxiety and perturbations about what was right or wrong, being judged by others, listening to the imposter syndrome, or falling into mental traps that sabotaged my peace of mind, I resolved to focus solely on my goals and move forward without looking back. This newfound sense of joy provided me with a firm foundation to immerse myself in my insights, to remain flexible, and to embrace the transformative power of the process.

Did this resolute behavior work all the time? The answer was both yes and no. Yes, it worked when my diet provided ample carbs and I had the luxury of rest, a precious commodity during the prolonged preparation. No, it did not work when I grappled with hunger in a calorie deficit, and my mind played tricks on me about food, leaving me unable to think clearly or make resolute decisions.

Chapter 9: Slammed.

The bittersweet symphony of life is such that we strive desperately to cling to what we can control, and only if we can control are we at peace and believe it is the conventional state of living. But what happens when you get slammed not in one direction but in various directions?

Well, you move on and never lose sight of your goals. The path to reach your goals is exceptionally long like a meandering road that has many stops, detours, deviations, roadblocks metaphorically speaking of course, and we all face these situations in many aspects of our lives. There are simply two ways to combat that: Fight or Flight.

Cliché as it sounds these words "Fight or Flight" the choice and the decision on how we react to the said situations makes all the difference. Frankly, there is never an enjoyable time for anything, you just must suck it up and do what you got to do. I was slammed, like a pile of bricks landed on my face and I had to find the hardiness to sort out the bricks and make a path to move forward.

The dawn of every new day is not automagically a positive start to the day. The news was intense with so many issues the world was facing together, people suffering and the Virus spreading like wildfire, controversial debates on how effective the mask is, even conspiracy theories of the Virus being a farce leading to people not adhering to protocols and thus the death rates on the rise.

I came across news that NPC competitions scheduled in the current month were cancelled due to state mandates of avoiding social gatherings and my thoughts would go down the rabbit hole of what would happen to my show in August. Sometimes I would console my rumination with a detached approach. Many weeks had passed, and I had come so far in my fitness journey. The sleepless nights, the burn in my core and my resolve put to the test time and again had taken a toll in my body for sure and my mind that had been challenged in this infamous year 2020, I still lived, thrived, to see the light of yet another day and to conquer yet another day. Sometimes optimism can be sabotaged with the influence of the environment around that was mostly negative in nature and anybody for that matter can be driven to deep down doldrums. Foreboding can grow manifold especially if you have become a hermit in your own home.

Tasks pile up, working from home, taking care of the home, family and my own needs, the unconscious bias of the sport looming every now and then which can bring down the morale and foreboding can grow and tire you. During days that needed affirmation, I told myself that I would be in acceptance if my show cancels at least I have a healthy mind and body as an outcome and learnt the art of healthy dieting and working out and on the same note, I wanted to walk and grace the stage, finish Strong this accursed prep that I felt sometimes had no end. I had to consciously reconnect, refresh, and recalibrate my thought process, from time to time to keep going with the daily activities. I had to be a beacon of hope for my kids who looked at me for strength, happiness, peace, and food. It all adds up, piles up, little by little to consume you and the efforts to lather, rinse, repeat to push all the negativity away gets harder and harder. I tried my best to keep it all together.

I had to try to keep it all together, pain and change is inevitable but reacting to it is optional. Every single day was important for me since I was on a quest to achieve the impossible.

I had to reinforce these mind battles with continued meditation. Moreover, I did not want to quit now, I had gone too far, and I wanted to finish it. Shelter in place to stay away from the natural calamities of the world came with home life redefined as corona virus continued to fester like cancer. Setting aside all the troubles, I focused on practicing and perfecting posing, continued to walk in heels. Fumbling, balancing, practicing daily with the image that stared back at me from the mirror, confidence grew within. I attended posing classes every week and I witness in the mirrors standing with other women, I belonged here. I was one of them, the making of a first-time body builder.

My inhibitions were dying all though there was a certain amount of risk involved amidst others in the posing class, I always had my mask on and even with my mask I could not mask feeling confident, bold, and had my chin up high during the practice. I even felt a sense of liberation to remove my shirt to show on what I have worked. I was no longer afraid to be in a Bikini outside the safety of my bathroom, I was posing in front of others, showing the best of my musculature and I was proud of myself, I felt like a winner against all odds.

Bodybuilding was truly an American sport, and I was not just the only one. Surrounded by so many bodybuilders in the making, I felt enthused and could easily forget about all the impediments that conspired to slow me down and would float through my moves, I was getting better in posing all though I had a long way to go.

I felt "American" to the core and that was a darn good feeling. True to the American culture, Americans accepted body building so easily.

Americans I interacted with in social media or at my workplace did not lift their eyebrows or condemn me like my Indian counterparts would have. Bodybuilding was welcome in my circle of interaction because all I received was good wishes and adoration for choosing a tough goal to achieve in their eyes. The environment we live in is so influential to your mindset and your goals. I had to surround myself with these like-minded people to keep going.

Strong Nation started providing the instructors Virtual training offerings to build our skills during the times when gyms were closed. This involved opportunities to get certification with NASM Group Fitness training, fighting elements, KATA basics, Social Media foundations where material was given to us to study and learn and then take an exam to become certified in various fitness areas.

In the personal development front, I made use of the resources that my workplace provided including getting virtual training on Change Management, Women of the world continued education, Thriving during crisis and many more for my intellectual stimulation. I let go of my old ways, dogmas, cultural restrictions, keeping my mind and body busy learning new things. I felt genuinely like a warrior with tenacity and gung-ho.

With my biweekly check-ins, I had increased pressure to lose body fat percentage goals. I was at 50 grams carbs for the day which was barely enough to keep my energy levels up. But I continued to slay with my workouts. Mornings before sunrise were always a blessing since I have always been a morning person getting out of bed with gusto. I would put on my headphones and binge watch Netflix while I ran intervals on the treadmill followed by one slice of Ezekiel Bread with six egg whites were a challenge for refuel. I tried to trick my brain in making the French toast with one slice and cutting them into small pieces so I could take longer to chew and hoping that gave me a false sense of fullness. I switched to Pam Spray that was zero fat for cooking, ate a lot of vegetables to fill the gnawing hunger that was becoming my close companion.

I continued to cry when it was time to feast on Gourmand cheat meals over the weekend. It was the same: Pizza and Tiramisu until the pressure of losing body fat became more prominent; I switched to making carb rich meals for cheat meals until Bony gave me the horrifying news that within the last 4 to 5 weeks there will not be any cheat meals. I savored them because I knew they would be taken away from me. Through the guise of time affluence, I was losing touch with my emotions. My sense of smell heightened, temptations of food provoked me from time to time, and the light headiness' was more frequent. The burning sensation at night came into resurgence with a constant reminder that I was depriving my body of much deserved carbs, followed by weakness to get through the day. The same level of protein kept me alive enough to continue my training, whether rain or shine. There were days I had to do two cardio sessions and I took my workouts to the great outdoors. Working out was a compulsion to keep breathing.

When it rained, I would complete HIIT workouts on the front porch that had a roof. Rain, thunder, lightning as my audience gave me an opportunity to be in tandem with nature, the connection of an ever-changing world and I was an agent of change. Although I started to move in a feeble and unsteady way I would continue working out. Working outdoors, I could mix up many ways of cardio at the end of the day. I could no longer practice my routines with StrongNation but took to biking and swimming. Nature did have healing powers and the connection was strong. Very soon I knew that my physical strength was spiraling down. I had lost weight, body fat and during weightlifting, I could not lift heavy anymore. I had neither power nor strength to do any PRs, if I could barely do four sets of fifteen reps without dying was a great achievement. Weightlifting or any resistance training was an uphill challenge, there were times I would cry during a leg curl because of the burn and the conflict of my mind to finish that one last rep that would make all the difference.

My family was incredibly supportive and knew the challenges that I was facing extremely well since they were seeing me struggling through them. My boys were in their best behavior to not push mom's "hot buttons" otherwise there would be catastrophic results. The world outside my world was still in a major pandemic and the continental United States soared with the highest Corona Virus infected rate. Florida was among the highest impacted states for the Virus.

Doctor offices were closed and opened only for virtual visits, hospitals overwhelmed, medical personnel overworked, scientists working day and night for a cure, political debates on the cause and effects of the Virus and so much more that was leading to a once in a century global disaster and here I was building my body, accepting changes within in and outside of my being and moving towards more changes with seriousness and sobriety. At least I was in control of my actions and was adapting to the external stimuli with my goals, or at least I thought I was, when the check-ins changed from biweekly to weekly.

Weekly check-ins resulted in more changes to my diet and exercise routines. I always had so many questions during my check-ins about this physiological body that was changing at a rapid rate, now I stopped asking questions, I just followed instructions. I was at peace that there were certain things that I could control but I was not able to anymore with even my diet nor my workout regimes that were changing I began to go with the flow.

I learnt firsthand to embrace the process and you will become it. Reactions, flight, or fight responses just lead to chemical imbalances which would raise cortisol levels, so it is best to let go, become a machine completing one task after another, whatever I was hit up with. It worked! Progress was uncanny, I was void of emotions, ignorant of the negativity of the world, all I could cognize was sweat, heart beating and rush of endorphins and blood flow that was necessary for my sanity check. I felt alive and that was all I needed to get me through the day.

Slammed as I was in in many directions, I continued to miss my bestie, but the long silence made me realize that I had deliberately volunteered her to share and support my fitness goals and journey, even if she did not understand it. What transpired between us was neither of our faults; I missed her and was waiting for the competition to complete so I could talk to her. I continued to post on social media and that was my connection, my support system, and empowerment. Bony continued to be my "text me a friend" my sounding board and I could vent out to her without any pride or prejudice, and she would listen, she could relate, and she knew exactly what to say to pacify me.

Lilyan was Bony's friend, a fellow coworker at my company and thus started a budding friendship. We chatted over texts so furiously since we wanted to know each other, and then I particularly wanted to know all her experiences as a two-time body builder. It is amazing how two people can connect, support, and empower each other when they have the same passion. Lilyan with her honest candor and sent by God, provided per perspective of body building, the aftereffects and the next shock that was waiting for me since I was nearing my goal with the pass of every day.

Peak Week!

Chapter 10: Peak Week, Deplete and weak.

A little over two weeks remaining from the competition date. I had reached my goal weight but was still struggling to reach my body fat percentage goal. At this point, I was performing three workouts in a day. Fasted cardio in the morning which was down to interval training on the treadmill with the emphasis to burn the fat, which was not budging at my abdominal area, coming down to fighting with the genetic makeup of my body at this point. I could not run continuously anymore. Weight training continued to traumatize me, because I could barely finish the sets and reps even if I reduced the weights. Weightlifting felt like a herculean task and left me feebly and almost wheezing for breath. But I carried on with my workouts just so I could check it off daily with no leeway for self-care, rest or recovery followed by the second cardio after weightlifting that involved going for a long walk outside or riding my bicycle in the neighborhood.

Due to low carb diet and prolonged calorie deficit with over training my brain started getting foggy when I realized I was having trouble remembering what set or what rep I was at during weight training.

It also started when I was on the bicycle biking around in the neighborhood if I was into be on the right side of the road or the left side of the road. I did not think of it much at that time, most importantly I was concerned about my light headedness that was becoming more recurring. Coach said it is due to low sodium in my diet and he recommended that I sip Powerade or BCAAs throughout the day and that helped.

I practically lived now in my workout clothes and felt guilty if I lacked movement due to working from home, or if I had to rest. Rest was restless, so I forced myself to watch brainless television so I could be tunnel visioned and would not move. I still had to follow my diet, but I stopped feeling hungry, as if my insides were dead.

The hormones Ghrelin (responsible for hunger) and Leptin (responsible for satiation) were MIA. I had to force feed at times and the other times I could not even tell I was hungry, or it was time to refuel until I started to eat and then I would feel like I needed to eat more. My cheat meals had stopped two weeks ago, and I could tell the difference immediately.

Before the cheat meal over the Sunday afternoon would fuel me until Wednesday before I would start feeling hunger pangs and exhaustion. But now, it was downright depressing, nothing to look forward to on Sunday afternoons, exhaustion, tiredness was tottering around me. To make matters worse, when my family would order food delivery and sit at the dinner table to eat, I would feel sad and angry about what my life has been reduced to. The aromatic smell of freshly cooked meal, the carb rich freshness was unbearable for me that I used to go elsewhere in the house so I could not hear, smell that gourmand that was consumed.

My world consisted of Eggs of all forms: Boiled, raw eggs, egg white cartons. I craved carbs; I craved sugar to get me through the day. Meditation kept me sane through these cravings and insanities I began to experience. Meditation made me realize that everything in this world is impermanent and change is part of life. Meditation reminded me that change, even this transformed body is not permanent, and I could not be looking this perfect all the time and I would change again. Then there were many more instances during meditation where I found myself dozing off in deep slumber with my neck bent down and my shoulders drooping in a weird way, and I would not even know when I drifted off into a dreamless state of mind. The feelings and hardships that I was going through would change too, and then there would be a day after the show when I could eat anything and everything I wanted to. Visions of Kaju Katli (Indian cashew and milk based sweet), ice-creams, tiramisu, pizza and all the treats you find in near the cashier section at a grocery store I could eat, and it would be all worth it.

I had become very lean, and my abdominal muscles were showing all the time. The area near the abdominal muscles had shrunk and shriveled reminding me of the metamorphous that I made my body go through. I started touching myself when I spent a lot of time in front of the mirror at this new self that was looking back at me to believe that I was changing and transforming. It was still summer months in Florida and was sweltering hot and humid outside, but I became cold. I was always cold due to dangerously low body fat that was continuing to go lower by the day.

I walked around in socks and hoodie, slept under two blankets as early as 6pm and would not budge till the alarm clock woke me up in the morning for my fasted cardio. I had changed drastically. My physical structure knew pain, endurance, resilience and recovery and my mental structure had matured in so many ways. Apart from the value of life, a home, family, nothing mattered to me.

Not the virus or any drama. My family became very accepting and compromising with me, the acceptance was mutual.

I thought of my bestie very much during my workouts and realized that she was voluntold to support and encourage me with this goal of bodybuilding which she would not get it, understand, or comprehend the complexity that was involved. I missed her terribly and was looking forward to talking to her after the show. I had cut her off for the very first time in my life and realized that I could manage my strength of wellbeing and decision making without her, I became independent.

My mind was pure but could not handle complexity. My mind was sensitive to the changing environment, and I could see knowledge in everything. I realized the repercussions of the chain reaction that sets off with the kind of input we give our bodies and mind and the consequences of it at a basic level such as what happens to our bodies when we eat unhealthy food vs. healthy food. The importance of strength training for sound joints and serving as protection to the organs within, especially as you age, more reason you must lift heavy things. I realized the importance firsthand of having a balanced macro meal, keeping protein steady, sufficient carbs and fat and to throw in abundance of vegetables of all colors to have a well-balanced, healthy meal.

What happens when we expose our minds to bad stimuli vs. good stimuli? The input and the output and the results that make each of us so unique in this world were an epiphany for me. Trusting the process had become a detox in my physical and mental progress and I was emerging as a different version or rather the best version of me. The time had come to buy my Competition Suit. With my online searches, I was flummoxed with what was the right bikini for me. As small as that contraption was, the array of styles and colors that were available online was interesting and amusing that I would be getting into one of them soon.

Walking the stage in front of an audience, with nothing to hide but only to show the progress I have made through these torturous months and flaunt it like a rebel was my finishing line. With my coach's recommendation, I made an appointment to visit a former body builder who makes competition suits that are NPC/IFBB approved. My husband and I drove to her house after an hour-long drive. A masked lady greeted us, and we were directed upstairs where the room opened to a massive bikini Ville. There were pictures on the wall of women with awards and sculpted bodies, bikini suits of all shapes and sizes hung everywhere. I tried the first few suits and fell in love with my reflection. The suits were shiny, glittery, and so sassy that I looked like the folks in social media, bold, beautiful, and able to carry out the tiniest of bikinis. I could not believe it when I saw the pictures my husband took of each suit, so I could compare, contrast, get second, third, fourth, opinion before I purchased the suit. Honestly and not so modestly speaking, all the suits fit me well and got out the best features in me.

If I had it my way, I would buy them all. After much deliberation, I narrowed the choices to three suits and finally purchased an expensive but beautiful turquoise sequin studded silky and shiny suit.

The top was lined with glittering silver, with shades of green and streaks of turquoise on them, and the bottom had the same positive aspect as sequins, strings to hold the bottom in place and just enough to show the backside glute definition.

To accessorize I purchased a silver studded fashion jewelry bracelet, fingering, and matching earrings. We were driving home with a small package filled with my arsenal that was also the most expensive piece of garment I ever got. I was prepared and ready now to strike a pose! Posing on the other hand practice was suffering, I knew the importance of posing but after passing each day, three workouts, working from home, preparing my meals I had no energy left to bring out the confident sexiness within me. The last thing I wanted to do was to put my heels on and do the walk! I tried but there was only so much I could accomplish successfully in each day.

It was like a conspiracy that once I was ready, the low carb brain fog kicked in to stay permanently.

The fog became denser when I entered Peak week just as Lilyan had told me. Mentally I was a mess, physically I was weak but overall, this corporal structure that I worked and slayed for looked rocking.

Cardio was not complete if I did not feel dizzy and my world was spinning, I had lost my appetite or I was hungry all the time, I could not tell the difference anymore. Peak Week had more plans in store for me.

Tottering to my check-in, the coach and I talked. I was exhausted physically and mentally now, I could not feel myself anymore, all the battles that I had had to face in the last twenty-five something weeks finally were catching up with me, taunting me to stop. But Peak week was here, I had to drag through it. What is peak week anyway, in summary it is carb loading, salt and water manipulation to get the perfect stage appearance?

Sounds easy I thought, but on the contrary, it became tougher to get through a day, to cook my meals, and to have a decent conversation with my family let alone working out and keeping up with the training.

I felt climbing the stairs was difficult without heavy breathing or asthmatic symptoms. I was confused and going through heavy ketosis. Not able to focus or concentrate with the recurring light headedness I decided to take time off from work for the entire week.

Time off from work is always a valuable gift, and this time I valued it more than ever.

My sole purpose of the time off was to check and recheck my stage bag, and everything that I had to be ready for the competition.

Pulled through with my daily workouts that had changed drastically which at this point I had no energy and did not care much on the quality of my work out if I could get through it and check it off for the day. My coach had said all my workout will end on Wednesday so I can rest up for the show.

My meals were changing by the day. At one point I was eating thirty-four egg whites in a day, and I was sick of eggs, I tried to make it in diverse ways using different spices to stuff it in and just get through the day. Then it got challenging when my coach said not to put salt in my food, so there is no water retention and I felt disgusted to eat the meals and wanted to starve instead. I had to force feed meals into my system so that I would not pass out and as it is, my light-headedness was happening many more times now. I gulped down water which was now one and a half gallons. I was eating sugar free Jell-O after every meal which was a redeeming quality.

I realized that normally, which seemed like eons ago, I have and many of us for that matter, have abundance of food around us all the time. The audacity of our attitudes towards food is pathetic, sorry to say. Food is considered entertainment, an object of abuse and criticism, a celebration, an addiction to cravings and hatred and a definition of who we are and what we like and dislike and here I was reduced to nothingness to consider food as fuel primarily. This was new to me, the ketosis was strong on me, my body was in a state of hormonal shock, and I could not take it anymore.

Trance like sluggishness loomed, my brain was weak to cognize, my breath was heavy and harsh, the weights I lifted had lowered in weight, and Pink Floyd's Dark Side of the moon playlist in the background was a perfect stance for a drug life dopey effect of my mind and body.

My body and mind were living but in a weird surreal state, never in my life have I felt so comfortably numb, which was also one of Pink Floyd's songs that made so much sense, the music the beats, the lyrics, and my situation. On the other hand, drinking almost two gallons was easy as I live in Florida and it is always hot with 360 days summer and five days winter, but the number of trips to the bathroom was getting me. I felt I should just live in the bathroom and thank the lord, toilet paper was not scarce like it was during the beginning of the pandemic, the supply chain had thrived and changed since then, and we had substantial amount of toilet paper at our disposal.

On the bright side of my ketosis and suffering was the image I saw from the mirror. I had lost all body fat and had essential fat remaining. My abdominal muscles were taut and showing six pack very clearly, my arms and legs had lines everywhere to show the bulge of what was left as muscle with my extreme diet.

The competition suit which normally I would find bold, sexy, and so revealing now fit me perfectly.

The suit looked as if it was tailor made for me. I remembered my coach and his words when I first met him.

Fitness and diet can change the health of a person and make them look good in clothes. But body building sport is such that you cannot hide anything, you need to have sculpted the body perfectly not to look skinny, or fluff but exactly right with musculature to show contours and grace. I practiced my posing in front of the mirror in perfection and was fascinated by the metamorphism that I saw. Months that felt like forever of training and dieting, were culminating to an end. I never looked like the image that I was seeing in the mirror ever in my entire freaking life. I was the best version ever, the perfect tailor made, stage ready first-time body builder! I was a winner, I smiled, and my eyes imploded with the hardships, dedication, discipline, emotional roller coaster experiences that I had endured and pushed my limits to lead to this celestial body. I had changed, inside and outside and emerged as a stronger and resilient woman. I had learnt and adapted how to lead a healthy lifestyle, the importance of food and exercise. I had tremendous respect for body builders now, going through the prep of how hard body builders work to transform into celestial bodies and push human limits and I was now one of them. I was reborn as Iron Chic.

The transformation is mind blowing. With the glittering suit, strutting on four and half inch's stiletto which by the way I was able to walk gracefully maybe not mastered I portrayed a stoic personality. Wednesday came at last, and I completed my last workout victoriously. I felt impaled yet imprisoned that I need not workout anymore. I did not want to lift weights, it traumatized me, sore, overstrained. I did not have to get up early in the morning and run on the treadmill anymore and as it is my right leg was hurting, I was in pain, every time my husband massaged me on my right leg, I would cry. Fantasies of what I would do post Show Day were planned in many ways and went through repeatedly in my mind.

My fantasies included eating food, normal food, not prep food, especially loads and loads of sugar and carbs and not feeling guilty or worrying about my check-ins. I would have energy to focus on my relationship with my husband and take care of my kids. I would be in control of what I eat and when I eat. I would binge watch Netflix, eat greasy pizza that I missed and top it off with a fat rich tiramisu, get fat, lose my abdominal muscles but be happy and live happily ever after. Trivial things but I missed and cherished and valued them now. Sometimes I could not believe that things would change, and I can relax and enjoy the lockdown benefits for working from home.

Thursday came with the crabs and suddenly I felt alive. It was a magical experience, carbs in my blood. My mind started working again; thinking clearly and the fog had lifted.

I was excited and now looking forward to the show. Although apprehensive about what Saturday Show had in store for us. The pandemic was still in effect, Corona Virus had reined humankind and alike, there were strict protocols to wear masks and to practice social distancing. The world was in turmoil, but the show must go on.

I checked the NPC website repeatedly to make sure that they had not cancelled the show. I was afraid of that, I wanted to grace the stage, finish this off strong. It would be the first time that we would be leaving the kids at home.

Then I packed my meals that were specific for the stage show needs. Lately my coach had changed my meals and adjustments of macros drastically and daily that I had to look repeatedly at the emails that he sent daily to ensure that I was following the diet. Then when I packed the measured meals, I was constantly getting confused of what meal was for which time. I finally put them in zip locks with meal number and date so I would not get confused. Amidst all the challenges of the day, my thoughts lingered to my best friend, I missed her, I wanted her so badly in my life now, but we were in different worlds, cultures, and I decided that now would not be the time to reconcile. I had to wait until the show was complete and then I would talk to her like I promised.

I cross checked everything once more that night before going to sleep. Friday, I had so many things to do for a change. The next few days would be sensational I thought. All the challenging work would be rewarded. I was rewarded already, looking at myself and the transformation that I went through. Walking the stage was an icing on the cake. I was tired but content with having carbs in my last meal, and I slept peacefully.

Friday morning, I woke up with a spring action from bed. Today was the day I become pretty or start to look pretty with self-care.

Since I had practically lived in workout dry fit clothes, it was a welcome change to wear carbon black liquid leggings that hugged my lower body and emphasized my slim waist, and a sleeveless crop top that accentuated my strong depleted arms that now showed muscles and no fat. The top precariously lingered just enough on my waist to show my abs. Normally I would never pull such an outfit off with my abdominal fat falling over leggings, but this was a peak week that I endured and survived. Although salt less food was my fuel, my water intake was now reduced to just a few sips and that had dehydrated me. The trick was to start with two gallons all week so that the body works hard to keep flushing out the water and the toxins that would become second nature only to trick the body to keep flushing fluids and toxins off the body even when I stopped hydrating the last two days. Science was used in peak week to look the best. I was stumped and stunned at this process when I heard of it firsthand and saw the results happening.

I had appointments all day long taken well in advance. With a mask on my face, and a prayer to the lord requesting corona virus would stay away from me. I was driving towards the beauty salon near my house to get my eyebrows threaded, preened, and shaped. It was weird to have the mask on all the time and the eyes had to show more than my words.

I felt suffocated to cover myself this way for this long and this was just the beginning. After my eyebrows were shaped, I drove to the hairdresser's salon for my next appointment: Hair.

Six months of being at home, eating right and hydrating well, my hair was thick, and long. I went through a nice package of shampoo wash that felt blissful after all these months of challenging work, and then treated my hair to an expensive hair package that included coloring, glossing, and styling to perfection. Sitting back getting my head massaged when my hair was washed, I felt like a queen. I felt I do so less to take care of my being; I valued and intended to continue self-care after the show.

The result was smashing! I had a great body already and now I had the good looks with Bollywood silky, shiny, voluminous long straight salon hair. Then with a rumble in my stomach as it was time for my third meal, I drove to the nail salon place for my next appointment, and they were waiting for me.

Things had changed in the world as I knew it that day; it was my first day out after an exceptionally long time. People moved around in masks, which looked funny, as if humans were under some sort of restraint or punishment not to speak and not to interact with other humans. The masks were of satirical variety on people I observed.

Masks on people around me were ranging from dull black to graphics, to designs and flashy colors. Humans adapt, life goes on, with or without Corona Virus looming in the air ready to kill someone. The nail place had changed too, there were translucent screens for each seat where I could get pedicure and manicure done, so that there is no direct contact of air or water droplets facing each other. I felt safe and carried a hand sanitizer with me and used it before and after every appointment.

There were other things in life outside of fitness, prep, measured macros and the feeling and experience of indulging in self-care to look like a star felt like a reward even during a pandemic. I came home ravenous but looking like a glamour model and my family, especially my husband, was in love with me all over again. He praised my hair, my eyes, my nails and toes and the salon look that I portrayed. With his help, I quickly posed for pictures as I knew I want this day to be memorable, and treasured for generations to come and stories to be told of a lady of Indian origin and the first lady in my family who became a body builder and achieved the toughest goal she ever could. I was a winner, and the day was going fantastic for a change. The crabs held, the fog lifted, I was excited.

Lugged my suitcase and my icebox filled with more salt less food in zip locks, kissed my boy's goodbye with a siren of instructions to lock the doors, not open the doors for anyone, to eat in time, to do their homework, go to bed at a sane hour. My husband and I were driving on the freeway towards the Hotel in Orlando where the show was to be held.

We talked about the kids like we always do when we are alone with each other's company.

My thoughts abated when we parked the car and took our suitcases into the hotel lobby. We had to secure our masks before entering since the state required it as mandatory for our protection. Inside, our temperatures were checked, and we had been banded on our wrist and we checked in to the room. My husband and I felt good to be outside of home, it felt like a mini gateway.

My husband relaxed on the bed after a long stressful week. I on the other hand had to unpack the icebox and put my precious zip locks in the mini fridge. I checked the watch, and I had enough time to gobble my meals before I had to go for my check-in and registration.

Removed the salt less egg white zip lock and gobbled it telling my husband that it tasted so bad, but it was so good for me today, cleaned up and grabbing my bag, my husband and I went to the second-floor ballroom where the registration was to be held. I did not have to try to look for the place where I had to check in, I just followed the place where I saw very fit people gathered. The feeling was such that I was walking into a world of extremely muscular, ripped, buffed, and sculpted people. Although they were all masked and dressed, it was so obvious how these walking sculptures were showing their hard work through their clothes. My husband and I were awed, surrounded by a distinct set of human species. We exchanged knowing glances at each other as we stared at everyone around us. I was supposed to be one of them and now I knew how tough this competition would be.

With no knowledge of what to expect or what I was supposed to do and coming out of quarantine for the last six months had short circuited my abilities to be relax but I stumbled through the process of registering and receiving a temporary NPC card, checking in with my weight, height and picking up my stage number badge and the free goodies that were offered to the contestants. Then my phone buzzed alerting me that I needed to rush to my last appointment for the day: Tanning.

I have never had any experience in tanning, but thanks to my bodybuilder friends, they had honestly and candidly prepared me for this. But knowing and experiencing are two distinct aspects and as much as I was mentally prepared, I was not really, and I went through this unique experience like a klutz and live to tell the tale. I signed my name verifying the appointment time at the desk in front of a ballroom and a tattooed and amazingly tall and lean lady asked me to go inside the ballroom. I opened the door and as the door automatically retreated to a close, my jaw automatically opened in a state of shock at the sight that beheld me.

All around were celestial bodies stripped down to nakedness and I was going to be one of them too. I was instructed by another woman to a kiosk and was told to remove all clothing and put it in a pile on the table and wait inside the open kiosk until called.

I felt cold as I stripped down completely and folded my dark colored full arm t-shirt and dark colored loose joggers. Never in my wildest dreams have I done this openly with people around me.

It was hard not to look around me as I waited to feel the cold draft touching my skin; women were all naked around me. Some women were already tanned, some were waiting to get tanned, some were standing still with their eyes on the ground, and others were tanned and putting on their clothes or checking their phones and heading out the door.

If there was a place where God created women carefully to perfection, grace, curves, flowing with smooth femininity and sexiness, it would have to be this place where I was. A sense of appreciation and celebration of life permeated within me to be part of this creation of womanhood. I was in the inner sanctum of woman who had pushed their limits, cried buckets, endured torture and hardships to emerge into the best versions of themselves. Each one of these women including me were lost to find themselves and what they are capable of and exulted to be souls of steel. It felt like a place in fantasy stories, like the Themyscira where warrior like powerful woman depicting strength, brawn, muscle, solidarity, Willpower gathered to form an elegant and dignified army to crush humankind. Woman were respecting the privacy of every other woman and not gawking or staring and I did the same. We were all in this together, we were an army of Iron Maidens, and body building was now our religion.

It was my turn, and I was instructed to step into another kiosk and another woman took a long powerful shower head and asked me to lift my arms and chin up and close my mouth and she sprayed a cold spray which impaled my bare exfoliated skin, and I began to shiver. The lady then asked me to do a quarter turn and the shivering increasing since I was now facing a small fan to dry the spray tan when another burst was sprayed to my sides. I was instructed to face my back to her and do the back pose and I stumbled and immediately apologized saying that this is my first time getting tanned. The lady was patient with me and for her I was just another body that needed to be sprayed. After another quarter turn and trembling for heat, clothes, and lack of body fat, my teeth were chattering.

I was asked to go back to the first kiosk where I had piled up my clothes and over there, I was asked to wait and dry in front of a small fan that was now blowing hard before getting dressed. Somewhere during this factory conveyor belt step-by-step process had hijacked my thinking. The worried tornado inside my head had faded and my heart was beating with a more fevered shaking in my legs. There is bitterness and pain in beauty, and standing there tanned among other tanned and non-tanned woman we are all the same, there is no questionable heritage, or cultural norms or restrictions. We were skinned to the way we intended to come into the world; we had organs and limbs, thoughts and aspirations clouded by emotions, now guided out of our heads and into our bodies. Microscopic values had been refashioned.

Dried, tanned and clothed I returned my thoughts to normal and walked out with a smile on my face with the experience that broke me for the better and looking forward to the yet to arrive dazzling stage experience. The rumble in my stomach and the thirst in my throat for food and water no longer affected me. I had an inner sense of resolve when I slept that night.

Chapter 11: Cinderella the Bodybuilder

The alarm buzzed at 4am Saturday morning August 15th which was the day India received Independence from the British rule in the 1900s. Eons after on this very day I woke up with a jolt, sprung in action with no food or water, brushed my teeth and lifted my shirt to show my tanned bare abs. Voila! I was depleted well, and drained off any excess water and all I could see were succinct defined six pack abdominal muscles. I tiptoed around the room, gathering my things, put on my mask and with great stealth I slipped out of the room careful enough not to wake up my husband. August 15th had arrived! I waited, and wondered about this day and it would also signify my independence from Prep, the training, and the extreme dieting that I had seriously followed for half a year along with an ankle injury that was screaming for rest and recovery. I would be free this evening, to eat up the world with my savage hunger!

My quest was going to reach its Zenith, I could fulfil my goal and break my prep tonight and celebrate. There would be no more fasted cardio, meal prep, weight training, check-in on progress, I will get my independence! But first I need to get pretty for the stage. My appointment for makeup was scheduled at 430 a.m.

The elevator, lobby, the hallways were so quiet and dark at this ungodly hour for a makeup session.

I looked at my phone again to ensure that my foggy brain had logged in at the exact time and I verified it was 430am.

I knocked on the door standing outside a dim lit hallway, half expecting no one to open it. My second knock was received, and a lady dressed in black leggings and a black shirt that was doing no injustice in showing the bulge of the muscle's underneath, opened the door and spoke.

"Hi, you must be my 430" she said cheerfully. I nodded and was escorted inside where there were tables that extended to the length of the room filled with makeup products arranged in a chaotic but organized manner. There were spotlights in vantage places where women in black robes were sitting in high foldable chairs with their eyes closed and like the lady who escorted me within were worker bees holding brushes, or makeup in their hands working their magic on the woman in black robes.

The worker bees or the makeup artists were all dressed in black with the company logo on their t-shirts. Narrow waists adorned with a band that had pockets to hold brushes, lipstick, and paraphernalia of cosmetic tools and essentials. It was a time warp in this room.

The place was bustling with activity and looked like a circus of sorts topped with fresh aroma of coffee in the air which reminded me of the familiar rumble in my stomach that was now my companion.

I could not drink water nor eat at this time, and I was directed to wait for instructions that my coach would send as to what I could eat before the show. For now, the aroma of Java beans in the air filled my nose and I enjoyed the feeling. One of the worker bees looked at me and gestured to me to take a seat on the highchair. I sat down and adjusted my legs and she looked at my face, forehead, eyes, cheeks, jawline and sipped her coffee. Her scrutiny was followed with questions.

"How are you hon."

"Good"

"What color is your suit hon."

"Turquoise blue" and I took out my phone to show her the color.

"Sit up straight, will ya?"

"What category are you competing in?"

"Bikini masters over 40+"

"First time?"

"How can you tell?"

She just smiled and spread out the foundation shades on the table nearest to me and got to work.

My stomach was rumbling, and an hour had passed. I was asked to sit straight, not move, turn to the right and stay that way, or lift my chin up and keep it that way, or just close your eyes and never open and finally, she smiled and gave me a mirror to see her creation. The face in the mirror was gorgeous, alluring, bewitching, captivating, divine, elegant, foxy, graceful, hype, inviting, lovely, magnetic, nice, pulchritudinous, ravishing, sublime, tantalizing, wonderful and many more words in my mental vocabulary came to me that very instant.

Walking back to the hotel room, I was ecstatic, the makeup was crowning glory, and all my appointments were done, I was ready for the show to begin. I opened the door to the room and my husband gaped at me in awe! I have been married to this man for eons, but it is always good to make my husband's heartbeat faster and lately I was doing that a lot with my transformation. A healthy relationship and lifestyle kept the romance going. I cannot complain as it just got better.

The much-awaited email flashed on my phone, as beautiful and surreal as my physical being had preened. I was but a dried-up beef jerky and a starving and parched savage within.

I was allowed to eat a bagel without any spreads and my husband was on the task to get me one.

I enjoyed the rush of dense carbs and gobbled it in no time. The rush I felt was euphoric, filled with energy and gait and the carbs were to pop my abdominal muscles out on stage. After taking a few pictures of my dazzling face and makeup and taking time to crop it well before posting on Instagram, so as to let my faithful followers who were supporting and encouraging my journey so far and reveling in self-affirmation of the almost immediate responses that poured in, I thought of my bestie.

Why was it so culturally wrong to compete in a body building state level competition? Why was it wrong to focus on the body and the beauty that evolved from my struggles and tussles to transform my body parts to the best of my ability down to my battles with my genetic makeup of my being? If I was doing wrong, why did I feel so much on top of the world, like a winner already even before the show? Why had my husband become so supportive through the prep and our romance had cranked up soaring high? Why didn't it feel wrong to me?

I felt like an American, respecting an American sport, and truly that was the reason! It was that simple!

I felt love for my bestie, I missed her terribly and wanted her to be a part of my experience, but it was not meant to be. For the very first time, I was freed and independent of my bestie's involvement and her acceptance of my actions. I could see myself differently now.

I was raised in India, but I grew into an adult in America, so my thoughts, my background, my experiences were culturally apart like day and night. There was no right or wrong in the matter and I knew it. I missed her.

I quickly texted her and told her I missed her and to wish me all the best and she immediately responded with her wishes. After the show I would talk to her, I was excited it had been months since I listened to her voice.

My husband reminded me that I had to get ready and go. I pulled out my clothes and slipped into the glittering competition suit and the sparkling jewelry. Within twenty-four hours of no water, I had depleted more, my tan was blended into my skin and the bikini was secured, my hair combed, and my lipstick touched up.

"Mirror mirror on the wall who is the leanest and strapping of all."

"My queen, the bronze body that you see is the leanest and strapping of all."

As if the fairy god mom cast a spell with her magic wand and made me a striking bronze body with lines, gracious curves, six pack abdominal muscles, prominent lats, biceps, triceps, juicy and perked glutes on well-defined hamstrings and quads.

I looked like a doll, a mannequin with salon hair, stage makeup, glittering bikini, tanned body standing on a four and half inch clear glassy heeled shoe.

I was preened and poised from what was left of me to become the best of me. I was Cinderella in every sense.

The conversation I was having with my image was spiritual. Six months of meal prepping five meals a day, drinking gallons of water, weightlifting, and fasted cardio sessions and undergoing peaking in peak week I stood tall, confident, bold, gorgeous, and exotic with musculature, charm and fatally and sexually attractive feeling an orgasm at my own self. I knew this was impermanent as is the nature of the world, everything changes, and it arises to pass away. Like fog that is thick and strong and impairs visibility but eventually the fog would clear, and reality will dawn. The process that I trusted and surrendered to was good to lead to a competitive stage, but it was not sustainable to have the lifestyle to continue and if it is not sustainable this quintessential body would not last long either. The lines would disappear, perfection would become imperfection, but I would be happy in my heart and soul to eat carbs and sugar! That is life, I guess!

Just like Cinderella this would be a magical experience after which I would be back in reality.

I was in acceptance of that feeling. Taking a few more pictures and practicing my posing routines I then wrapped myself in the long silk black body gown and felt that my waist was so tiny and delicate.

My husband and I settled in the great room where the competition would be held. The added height gave me confidence as I walked in. The great room was palatial, and the stage was lit up. Folks were trickling in now and it was interesting to observe the audience all looked fit and strong, or at least most of them. The bodybuilding industry was a whole unique experience for me as this was my first time. My husband and I sat down on chairs that were organized with social distance in mind and we were very occupied looking at people who have endured pain in battle to look like superheroes. I was in some tough competition for sure.

We were nearing Showtime and the PA announcement conveyed that all athletes are required to report backstage. I kissed my husband, and he wished me good luck and I made my way with my suitcase on my trails towards the backstage.

The backstage was crowded with contestants of all divisions. At first it looked chaotic to walk backstage trying to find my coach or someone I knew.

Then there were leads or volunteers who walking around with a pen and a pad and calling out names of contestants. I was instructed to get in line for the oil spray that was at the back corner from where I stood. I was referred to the competition number or badge that I was given during registration that was pinned to my bikini bottom. I had to walk backstage where I saw people ready in their suits, around me.

Women were clicking individual or group selfies and had shed their gowns and looked gorgeous in their competition suits. The bikini division had a certain make for suits so I could clearly see who was competing in my division and who was not. There were tanned women of all shapes and sizes who were busy preparing to get on stage. Some of them were taking their robes out, some applying makeup touchups with portable mirrors, some brushing their hair to remove the frizz. Some just sitting down and browsing on their phones. Some women were lined up to get to the stage entrance and were working with resistance bands to get that extra pump right before the stage appearance.

Men bodybuilders looked so formidable in their tiny suits that covered their glute areas so lovingly.

Men varied and personified personalities of Marvel superheroes with rippling mountains of muscles.

I thought to myself they do not need to worry about frizzy hair, or lipstick getting smudged due to wearing a mask, or worry about hormonal imbalances in menstrual cycles: Oh yes, that was a perpetual problem with the relentless nature of the prep, especially during peak week when the hormones go insane.

There were others who were oblivious of where they stood or who was around but they were deep in the thought process working their routines and poses in front of portable mirrors or phones placed at vantage angles so they could record their moves. Some of them were eating rice cakes or candy treats, to pop their abdominal muscles minutes before hitting the stage. It was a circus of sorts except instead of animals I was going through humans who shared the same DNA in the spirit of bodybuilding.

Finally, I caught a glimpse of my coach talking to a woman I recognized from my posing class and hurried towards them. I greeted my coach with a hug and acknowledged the others who were familiar to me all though I did not know their names when my stage number was called, and I was directed to stand in a line at the corner of the backstage to get oil sprayed on.

The show was going to start with the older division and work its way down to the younger age's divisions. The women in the line did not look over forty plus at all.

They had bodies that had many more lines than I did, muscles and curves that I never knew existed in the human being and much more clearly defined abdominal muscles than I was showing that I almost felt like I looked like a long thin lean stick compared to them. The feeling of confidence faded almost immediately along with the growing rumbling in my core and parched throat, I knew my energy reserves were low, but I had to keep going, finish strong.

I took off my robe folding it neatly opened the suitcase and placed it inside and removed the clear heels and put them on holding to the wall for support, my arch enemy had kept me accountable and I worked hard to walk in them and make them an extension of my legs but seldom I would lose my balance. With low reserves I felt light-headedness once more but supported and pulled myself up.

I needed to pull through when the world was spinning. It was my turn when I moved in the line and came in front of a lady who had glue in her hands.

Methodically she asked me to turn my back towards and she slid glue into my bikini bottom so it would not ride on the stage.

Then she turned and added glue to my bikini top, so it stayed in place and then I was ushered to step into the kiosk when a fresh tan/oil was sprayed on my triceps area and then lower part of my behind.

The concept was to highlight with a shine the muscles in this area when I pose on stage and the light would be shown brightly on my body. After a thorough sweep of the lady's eyes on every part and striation of my body, her expression changed to approval.

I heard my number immediately after I stepped outside the kiosk, and I was instructed to stand in line to get on the stage. Bodybuilding bikini expert's division (women 40+) and the show coordinators were busy checking off the names or the numbers on their pads and I was the 2nd to go up on stage. This was it. I barely had time to think and left my suitcase on the wall and wanted to go back to get my bands so that I could pump my muscles, but the coordinator was adamant that I should not leave. I desperately looked around and found a pair dumbbell on the floor which I grabbed and did some movements for my upper body so I could save that pump that would occur for the next few minutes.

The women in front of me and behind me looked like celestial goddesses from the fairy tales I grew up listening to as a little girl. If I had all the time in the world, being backstage, my linguistic quirks would have reached a level of creativity and literature of the perfect bodies with which I was surrounded.

With victory and glory, I stood waiting for my cue to go on stage. I was a winner already for having survived these last six months, against all odds in this insane year 2020. From shifting gears working from home, adjusting to domestic life, balancing act of family and career, the endless cooking, dealing with chronic self-doubt, mastering the balancing act of walking in four and a half inch heels, isolation and social distancing from the bizarre and outside the conventions and humdrum of routine life that was caused by Covid, staying alive with a deadly virus on the loose, being creative with home gym and fighting to be my authentic self-breaking cultural platitudes and value system and finding my way......I had come a long way.

My relish for fitness had kept me sane in this insane world. Here I stood in my element, with the decisive moment embellished with a bronzed tan, wearing a coquettish bikini and matching panoply of flashy jewelry.

All though my excitement and nervousness was more like hysteria, I was at the zenith of my prep and my head started to spin and I had to take a few breaths, close my eyes and tell myself "Don't pass out ....not now, pass out in a few minutes after, don't pass out".

I was hungry and thirsty, and I knew I could not afford to pass out now; I must finish this strong. My flurried chronicles disappeared when I heard my name called out. With my chin up, chest lifted, smile on my face, I walked into the middle of the stage with renewed energy as if the stage were like walking through a prism with a slice of power, promptitude, and renewed countenance to fulfil my quest.

What can I say about the experience! I walked with intention to the center of the stage, I could hear the crowds cheering me, I heard my name, and with fluidity I orchestrated my front pose with the brightest smile as I looked down at the judges one at a time. I could hear the music playing in the background and with immense mind muscle connection, got into the quarter turn and then the back pose paused to show my well-defined glutes before returning to the quarter turn transition as flashes of light moved on me and back to my front pose. Lifting my hand in a wave, I gave yet another smile to the judges and walked to the back of the stage to take my place while the next woman began her drill. Standing behind still in my pose, I was shivering, my legs were shaking, but I kept my smile .... I had done it. Like a protagonist who had set out on a quest and faced obstacles that I overcame in pursuit of this very goal right here, right now pierced my heart with enhancement. Every conundrum, everything faded away!

Just like Cinderella, at the stroke of midnight, the magic faded away!

Chapter 12: She lifts happily ever after

Did I go home with the trophy and medal that night?

I did not. NPC Mid Florida State level bodybuilding competition is not for the faint hearted and I had some severe cutthroat competition with woman in my division who scored better than I did in many ways. I was not vexed that I did not win. I was a winner for surviving the most challenging goal that I had ever embarked upon against all odds this year. I realized how tough bodybuilding can be but on the contrary, I emerged as a new person. I had grown mentally, physically, and spiritually through the process. That night, my friend, my inspiration, and the very person who introduced me to this sport had come to support me. Without inhibitions of Covid, social distancing, I hugged Bony, and I was in tears when she presented to me custom handmade cookies, and organic dark chocolate hazelnut candy bar. I could not stop eating when my husband, Bony, and I exited out the great room and to celebrate the hype and happiness of the entire experience.

I made Bony proud, I drove her insane with my constant texts when the clouds of doom were upon me during my prep, but she had patiently listened to me, walked my side at every step of the way.

When microscopic core values were challenged, she lifted me up and supported me day or night guiding and helping me through feast and famine, do or die, fight or flight difficulties that I went through. I had unfeigned admiration for her, I had found a best friend in her for life.

My family was incredibly supportive through the battles of course. My kids were in acceptance of my needs and shortcomings. My boys had grown with an image of mom who loves movement, dance, and strength training. They were privy of the fact that other mothers had manicured nails and I had ripped skin calluses. My husband loved me and my passion that he had gifted me a massive Everest punching bag for my birthday. He was accustomed to the fact that if he introduced anything fitness related, I would take it to extremes, like the time when he introduced me to StrongNation (formerly known as Strong by Zumba) I took it as a challenge and became a Strong Nation instructor after my first introductory class. Another time when he introduced me to weightlifting and BARBELL, I became so passionate about it that I became a State Level Body Builder. My husband would joke from time to time that he needs to be careful what he introduces me to, since I tend to go to the extremes with it.

Blessed as I was to have a battalion of sterling individuals, friends whom I would call family have supported me in my fitness passion through the years and I am in much heartfelt gratitude for them. Without these individuals I would not have been empowered, focused, or fit!

Donna was my ex-colleague at work who was totally into accumulating steps and being part of challenges in Fitbit. Donna's influence at work got me wearing a Fitbit and becoming more cognizant about movement during the day in corporate life. It was the times when my boys were young, and I was a supermom barely juggling family and career that Donna came into my life and pulled me to try out the Gym at work for a free month with her referral. That was my first introduction to the Gym, the temple of muscle and iron.

Here I met dynamic and most ingenious coaches/personal trainers Danny and Kelly who paved the way for growth in fitness.

The coaches trained me through every aspect from form, technique, agility, Tabata, weightlifting, HIIT and at the Gym is where I found my love for boxing. The flexibility to have a gym on premises where I worked helped to attend classes along with the balancing act of career and family. Through time my endeavors became passionate so that I was selected as a member of the year at the Gym which included having a blown-out poster of me placed in the Hallways of my office and I was known and famous because of this milestone.

It was through Donna and connection in Facebook that I learned about Bony who became a fabulous body builder, and my journey began with Bony, and my competition ended with Bony by my side. Lilyan was a ray of sunshine and optimism and having her come into my life at the right time and place was a blessing.

Lilyan filled in the gaps and became another robust friend whom I could lean on to get her perspective on her journey towards her competition goals.

I will always remember Lilyan's words that served as an anchor for the aftereffects of the competition that she shared with me.

Lilyan conveyed to me during our conversations and made me aware of the image of oneself after the show, the sheer nature of the prep and the not so sustainable lifestyle that I would lead which will eventually fade away the lines and curves and the perfect stage body away and reality strikes hard can mentally provoke and mess a person up. Her wisdom helped me prepare mentally for what was to come after the show, since I was so focused on everything that led to the show.

To all my StrongNation friends that I have come to love from the time I obtained my license and certification as a StrongNation instructor, you have always been so dear to me and I cherish all the fantastic times we have worked together in Sync labs, gym group classes when there was a world free of COVID. I loved and cherished all the time we were together dancing or performing plyometrics moves. I only have love for each one of you in my heart and look forward to many new experiences together.

Finally, my bodybuilding coaches Ty and Jo: the powerful, strong, down to earth, family friendly coaches who inspire and serve people to become the best version of them, I am so blessed and honored to have training with the dynamic duo. My frequent check-ins, meal plan and training changes and adjustments, to learning posing that was such a daunting task when I began and to emerge and spread my wings and become someone whom I thought I was not capable of. My eternal and astronomical gratitude for your coaching through the months is much appreciated. I enjoyed every experience good and bad becoming a Pope product to fulfil my quest and achieve an even greater aim.

Of course, there are many more Indian and American friends who are my well-wishers that I would be indebted who were pivotal for my success as well, and if I mentioned the names the list would go on and on.

My quest and why did I do this?

My god gifted parents introduced me to classical Bharatanatyam Indian dance and I grew up with limbs that craved for movement through the years.

A husband who had a wakeup call and transformed into a fit, strong, attractive, and powerful individual with the introduction of weight training, and the people I met who I learnt from lead to my quest.

The past and the present are inextricable; life goes on with the passing of day and night. Tumultuous and ludicrous this year 2020 has been with the pandemic, gave me an opportunity to accomplish, self-care to adapt a healthy lifestyle which made me realize that I have a thirst for challenges and growth and that is simply who I am.

Many months have passed after the show and my home has become my abode. My family and I are shut away from the world while we wait for the mass use of the vaccine that would provide us immunity to Covid 19. My day starts with the alarm that wakes me at 5am. I wake up, freshen up, put on my workout clothes and sneakers, and do 45 minutes of any form of fasted cardio. Through the day, I follow the five meal plans by eating every three hours a more relaxed macro meal of carbs, protein, and fat and in the evening, I lift weights in the heart of my master bedroom where the Smith machine that served me throughout the prep stands. On occasion I indulge in cheat treats and in between meals snacks and always hydrate drinking gallon water.

My stage body is what I will always compare myself to no doubt, even though I continue to transform building muscle and strength. Will I compete again in a body building competition?

When the world is free of the deadly virus, and I have forgotten all the impediments and hardships that I had to go through being a first-time body builder. But for now, I enjoy food, I enjoy sugar, I enjoy the energy and the capabilities I have gained, and I lift happily ever after.

THE END

We all struggle at times to adjust and adapt to the internal and external world. So have I personally faced and witnessed the turmoil of this wild concoction of a mind that I secretly hide from the world and the people around me, lest they might think me a weak maiden. Careful have I been in weaving a façade or an armor of strength, sustainability and dependability ensuring that I am portraying a powerful image in the eyes of my kith and kin. Thus, drawing my internal power reserves to keep the life source humming like a reliable and robust piece of machinery with zero defects.

Internalized as I am, thoughts are loud and clear that only I can hear. I have reached a certain singularly queer calm and fatigue with a chemical amalgamation that is both jarring and satisfying at the same time. The chord to the world is severed, the world is suffering, and it has turned its back on us and thus I shall turn my back on it. Exulted as I was when the connection was severed, giving me the gift of time to carve my path to goals to meet, promises to keep and to realize my dreams. Breaking through the social norms did I break through my internal resolve and evolved I must say with pride into a stronger, resilient, and beautifully attractive woman. Yes indeed, pay attention that is what happened during the pandemic when I took upon my heart and soul to become a first-time body builder. I bore the storm head on, fighting with grace and courage at what the source or the invisible force had in plan for me as impediments to overcome, to fall but to rise again from the scars and wounds becoming Iron Chic. This is my story of empowerment that I am willing to share and inspire you and make your reading pleasure worth your while.

Here are a few macro-based vegetarian meals that I experimented with and perfected during my meal prep. Please note that the macro measurements of carbohydrates, fat, and protein can vary for each person based on their daily caloric intake and body weight. Use your discretion wisely.

1. French Toast
2. Oats Pancakes
3. Schezwan Egg fried rice
4. Tofu Power bowl
5. Chickpeas Garlic rice
6. Egg Salad with cucumbers
7. Vegetable Egg Scramble / Oats upma
8. Potato cutlets
9. Power smoothie

Easy French Toast Recipe

Ingredients:

1. 6 slices of Ezekiel Bread
2. 6 eggs
3. 1/2 teaspoon cinnamon
4. 1/4 teaspoon nutmeg
5. Cooking oil spray
6. Walden Farms sugar-free jam or mixed berries for serving

Instructions:

1. In a bowl, crack the eggs and beat them until they are well combined.
2. Add the cinnamon and nutmeg to the beaten eggs and mix thoroughly.
3. Heat a non-stick pan over medium heat and spray it with cooking oil.
4. Dip each slice of Ezekiel bread into the egg mixture, ensuring both sides are coated.
5. Place the coated bread slices onto the hot pan.
6. Pour any remaining egg mixture over the bread slices in the pan.
7. Allow the bread to cook until the egg mixture begins to set and turn white.
8. Using a spatula, fold the edges of the egg mixture over the bread slices to cover them.
9. Flip the bread slices over to cook the other side until golden brown and cooked through.
10. Serve the French toast hot, topped with a dollop of Walden Farms sugar-free jam or with a side of mixed berries. Enjoy your delicious breakfast!

Simple Oats Crepes Recipe

Ingredients:
1. 1/2 cup oats
2. 6 egg whites
3. Pinch of cinnamon and nutmeg
4. 1 scoop of your favorite protein powder
5. Sugar-free maple syrup

Instructions:

1. In a blender, combine the oats, egg whites, cinnamon, nutmeg, and protein powder. Blend until smooth.
2. Heat a non-stick pan over medium heat.
3. Pour a portion of the batter onto the hot pan, swirling it around to spread it thinly into a crepe.
4. Cook the crepe for a few minutes until the edges start to lift and the bottom is golden brown.
5. Carefully flip the crepe and cook the other side until lightly golden.
6. Repeat with the remaining batter, making additional crepes.
7. Serve the crepes warm with a drizzle of sugar-free maple syrup.
8. Enjoy your delicious and nutritious oat crepes!

Easy Schezwan Egg Fried Rice Recipe

Ingredients:

1. 6 boiled eggs or 1 cup mashed tofu
2. 1/2 cup cooked jasmine rice
3. Chings Schezwan sauce
4. Finely chopped colored peppers
5. Finely chopped purple onions
6. Cut broccoli and cauliflower
7. 2 tablespoons finely chopped fresh basil
8. Finely chopped scallions
9. Salt to taste
10. Black pepper
11. Cooking spray or oil

Instructions:

1. If using boiled eggs, remove the yolks and chop the egg whites into small bite-size pieces. If using tofu, mash it and set it aside.
2. Heat a pan over medium heat and lightly coat it with cooking spray or oil.
3. Add the chopped veggies (colored peppers, purple onions, broccoli, cauliflower) to the pan along with a pinch of salt and black pepper. Sauté until the veggies are half-cooked. If the pan becomes dry, add a splash of water to prevent sticking.
4. Once the veggies are halfway cooked, add a spoonful of Schezwan sauce to the pan and continue cooking for another minute, ensuring all the veggies are coated with the sauce.
5. Add the cooked jasmine rice to the pan and stir-fry with the veggies and sauce on low heat for about a minute, ensuring everything is well combined.
6. Turn off the heat and sprinkle the chopped scallions and fresh basil over the rice mixture. Give it a final mix.
7. Serve the Schezwan egg fried rice hot and enjoy the delicious flavors!

Simple Tofu Power Bowl Recipe

Ingredients:

1. Medium firm tofu, cut into bite-size cubes
2. Spices: Coriander, Cumin, Garam Masala, Chili powder
3. 1 teaspoon finely chopped garlic
4. 1 teaspoon finely chopped ginger
5. Cucumbers sprinkled with paprika
6. Chopped vegetables: eggplant, celery, onion, spinach
7. Fat-free cooking oil spray
8. 1/2 cup cooked jasmine rice

Instructions:

1. Preheat your air fryer to 350 degrees Fahrenheit.
2. Toss the tofu cubes with a teaspoon of olive oil, salt, and pepper.
3. Place the seasoned tofu in the air fryer basket and cook for 5 minutes until golden brown and crispy. Once done, set aside to cool.
4. In an Instant Pot, combine the chopped vegetables, garlic, and ginger. Pressure cook on low for 8 minutes.
5. Allow the vegetables to cool slightly, then keep the pressure-cooked water (do not strain it all).
6. Add the air-fried tofu to the cooked vegetables in the Instant Pot to create a curry-like consistency. Mix well.
7. Serve the tofu and vegetable mixture hot over cooked jasmine rice.
8. Garnish with sliced cucumbers sprinkled with paprika for added flavor and color.
9. Enjoy your nutritious and delicious tofu power bowl!

Easy Chickpea Garlic Rice Recipe

Ingredients:

1. 1 cup cooked chickpeas
2. 1/2 cup cooked jasmine rice
3. Freshly minced garlic cloves
4. Chili flakes
5. Salt to taste
6. 1 teaspoon olive oil
7. Finely chopped cilantro
8. Juice of half a lemon

Instructions:

1. Heat a skillet over medium heat and add olive oil.
2. Add the minced garlic to the skillet and sauté until lightly browned and fragrant.
3. Sprinkle chili flakes into the skillet and stir to combine with the garlic.
4. Add the cooked chickpeas to the skillet, stirring to coat them evenly with the garlic and spices.
5. Reduce the heat to low and add the cooked jasmine rice to the skillet. Mix everything well to combine.
6. Cook the chickpeas and rice mixture for a few minutes until heated through.
7. Remove the skillet from the heat and transfer the chickpea garlic rice to a serving plate.
8. Garnish with finely chopped cilantro and squeeze fresh lemon juice over the top.
9. Serve hot and enjoy your flavorful and nutritious chickpea garlic rice!

Simple Egg Salad with Cucumbers Recipe

Ingredients:

1. 6 boiled eggs
2. Finely chopped cucumbers
3. 1 teaspoon sugar-free maple syrup
4. 2 teaspoons paprika
5. 1 teaspoon coriander powder
6. Salt to taste
7. Finely chopped cilantro (optional)

Instructions:

1. Peel the boiled eggs and discard the yolks.
2. Chop the egg whites into bite-size pieces and place them in a mixing bowl.
3. Add the finely chopped cucumbers to the bowl with the egg whites.
4. Sprinkle sugar-free maple syrup, paprika, coriander powder, and salt over the egg whites and cucumbers.
5. Gently toss everything together until well combined.
6. Taste and adjust seasoning if needed.
7. Optional: Garnish with finely chopped cilantro for added flavor and freshness.
8. Serve your egg salad with cucumbers immediately or refrigerate until ready to serve.
9. Enjoy your simple and delicious egg salad!

Easy Vegetable Egg Scramble & Oats Upma Recipe

Ingredients for Veg Egg Scramble:

1. 1 jalapeno, finely chopped
2. Colored peppers, finely chopped
3. Onions, finely chopped
4. Spinach, finely chopped
5. Salt and pepper
6. 6 egg whites or liquid egg whites
7. 1 teaspoon olive oil

Ingredients for Oats Upma:

1. 1/2 cup uncooked oats
2. 1 green chili, finely chopped
3. 5 curry leaves
4. 1/2 teaspoon chopped ginger
5. Cilantro, finely chopped
6. Salt to taste
7. 1 teaspoon olive oil

Method for Veg Scramble:

1. Heat olive oil in a skillet over medium heat. Add the chopped vegetables (jalapeno, colored peppers, onions, spinach) and sauté for two minutes.
2. Season the veggies with 1 teaspoon of salt and a sprinkle of water. Mix well, then remove from the skillet and set aside.
3. In the same skillet, spray cooking spray and pour in the 6 egg whites, spreading them evenly.
4. As the egg whites begin to cook and turn white, reduce the heat and use a ladle to scramble them. Once cooked, turn off the heat.
5. Mix the sautéed vegetables with the scrambled egg whites and serve.

Method for Oats Upma:

1. In a microwave-safe bowl, combine the chopped green chili, ginger, onions, and olive oil. Microwave for 1 minute.

2. Remove from the microwave and add the oats, salt, and enough water to cover the oats.

3. Microwave for 4 minutes or until the oats are cooked to your desired consistency.

4. Garnish the cooked oats upma with finely chopped cilantro and serve.

Enjoy your delicious and nutritious breakfast of Vegetable Egg Scramble and Oats Upma!

Simple Potato Cutlets Recipe

Ingredients:

1. Cumin, sea salt, garam masala, and chili powder
2. 5 ounces mashed potatoes
3. 6 boiled egg whites, shredded or chopped
4. Crème of wheat (semolina)

Method:

1. Pressure cook the potatoes until soft. Once cooked, mash them in a bowl and add the cumin, sea salt, garam masala, and chili powder. Mix thoroughly.
2. Add the shredded or chopped boiled egg whites to the mashed potato mixture. Mix until well combined.
3. Take portions of the mixture and shape them into patties of desired size.
4. Gently dust both sides of each patty with crème of wheat (semolina).
5. Heat a skillet over medium heat and toast the potato cutlets until golden brown on both sides.
6. Once cooked, remove from the skillet and serve hot with tomato ketchup on the side.

Enjoy your delicious and crispy potato cutlets!

Simple Power Smoothie Recipe

Ingredients:
1. 1/2 cup liquid egg whites
2. Chobani sugar-free yogurt
3. 1/2 scoop protein powder
4. 1 teaspoon sugar-free syrup
5. 1/2 cup oats
6. Ice cubes

Method:

1. In a blender, combine the liquid egg whites, Chobani sugar-free yogurt, protein powder, sugar-free syrup, oats, and a few ice cubes.

2. Blend the ingredients until smooth and well combined.

3. Pour the smoothie into a glass and enjoy your refreshing and protein-rich power smoothie!

Note: Feel free to adjust the consistency by adding more liquid or ice cubes as desired.